The Mental Health Professional's Guide to Managed Care

Rodney L. Lowman and Robert J. Resnick, Editors

American Psychological Association
Washington, DC

Published by
American Psychological Association
750 First Street, NE
Washington, DC 20002

Copies may be ordered from
APA Order Department
P.O. Box 2710
Hyattsville, MD 20784

In the UK and Europe, copies may be ordered from
American Psychological Association
3 Henrietta Street
Covent Garden, London
WC2E 8LU England

Typeset in Century Schoolbook by Easton Publishing Services, Inc., Easton, MD

Printer: Data Reproduction Corporation, Rochester Hills, MI
Cover Designer: Minker Design, Bethesda, MD
Technical/Production Editor: Mark A. Meschter

Library of Congress Cataloging-in-Publication Data
The mental health professional's guide to managed care / edited by
  Rodney L. Lowman and Robert J. Resnick
    p. cm.
  Includes bibliographical references and index.
  ISBN 1–55798–232–5
  1. Managed mental health care—United States. I. Lowman, Rodney
L. II. Resnick, Robert J.
  RC465.6.M46 1994
  362.2'045—dc20   93–47187
                                      CIP

British Library Cataloguing-in-Publication Data
A CIP record is available from the British Library

Printed in the United States of America
First Edition

Contents

Contributors

Carol Shaw Austad, Central Connecticut State University, New Britain, Connecticut

Robert W. Bottinelli, Private Practice, Margate City, New Jersey

Patricia M. Bricklin, Institute for Graduate Clinical Psychology, Widener University

Anthony Broskowski, Prudential Life Insurance Company of America, Roseland, New Jersey

Elizabeth Q. Bulatao, American Psychological Association, Washington, DC

Nicholas A. Cummings, American Biodyne, Inc., San Francisco, California

Patrick H. DeLeon, United States Senate Staff, Washington, DC

Leonard J. Haas, University of Utah Medical Center, Salt Lake City, Utah

Beatrice Harris, Harris, Rothenberg International, New York, New York

Shirley Ann Higuchi, America Psychological Association, Washington, DC

Rodney L. Lowman, The Development Laboratories, Houston, Texas

Russ Newman, American Psychological Association, Washington, DC

Beth Egan O'Keefe, Southpark Psychology, Moline, Illinois

Marilyn Puder-York, Private Clinical and Consulting Practice, New York, New York

Robert J. Resnick, Department of Psychiatry, Medical College of Virginia, Virginia Commonwealth University, Richmond, Virginia

Linda M. Richardson, The Development Laboratories, Houston, Texas

Gary R. VandenBos, American Psychological Association, Washington, DC

Introduction

Rodney L. Lowman

If you are a mental health professional practicing in today's delivery environment, you must be knowledgeable about managed care. This book is intended to help you learn to operate effectively within managed-care systems by explaining what managed care is, how it affects your mental health practice, and where the managed-care field needs to go next. Researchers will also find many relevant issues requiring their attention.

When the American Psychological Association's (APA) Board of Professional Affairs (BPA) first planned in the late 1980s a publication for psychologists on managed mental health care, relatively little was known or written about the subject. Since then, a number of articles and books, mostly practical coping guides for mental health professionals, have appeared (e.g., Austad & Berman, 1991; Committee on Managed Care of the American Psychiatric Association, 1983; Fitzpatrick & Feldman, 1992; Goodman, Brown, & Deitz, 1992; Sharfstein & Beigel, 1985). Now, with the publication of *The Mental Health Professional's Guide to Managed Care*, many of the more pressing substantive issues revolving around managed-care systems are addressed. Are mental health costs really as out of control as so many have contended? Are all forms of managed care the same? What has APA done about managed care? What have the courts had to say about it? How should mental health benefits optimally be designed? How does managed care affect the mental health professional's day-to-day practice?

This book is the result of a longstanding interest in managed care and in helping mental health professionals cope effectively with and influence such systems. It includes the initial BPA managed-care project (chapter 3), adding several chapters (1, 2, 4, 6, 7, and 8) that originally appeared in a special section in *Professional Psychology: Research and Practice* (see Lowman, 1991), and two chapters (5 and 9) that were specially commissioned to bring the book's treatment of the topic up to date. Although many of these chapters were written with an intended audience of psychologists in mind, the issues apply equally to all mental health professionals—psychiatrists, social workers, counselors, psychiatric nurses, and psychologists alike.

In chapter 1, Broskowski familiarizes readers with the financial pressures that have fueled (and continue to fuel) the managed-care movement. The history of managed care is outlined by DeLeon, VandenBos, and Bulatao in chapter 2. Chapter 3 (by Resnick, Bottinelli, Puder-York, Harris, and O'Keefe) defines the most prevalent managed-care systems, comparing and contrasting how they function and describing the issues that mental health professionals face within each system.

As any area of practice grows, a number of complicated legal and ethical issues emerge, and parameters for practice often must be reassessed. Newman and Bricklin (chapter 4) provide an overview of important legal and professional issues associated with managed care, and Higuchi (chapter 5) provides a state-of-the-art review of the rapidly evolving legal environment affecting managed care. In chapter 6, I provide extensive mental health benefit analyses of corporate data, which demonstrate cost problems and the financial effects of treating patients over time. Haas and Cummings (chapter 7) address the important ethical and professional practice issues that psychologists must consider before providing services through managed mental health care systems. Richardson and Austad (chapter 8) help practicing clinicians address true-to-life realities of professional practice in today's managed-care world. Finally, in chapter 9, I summarize critical synthesizing issues and next directions for managed care.

References

Austad, C., & Berman, W. H. (1991). *Psychotherapy in managed health care: The optimal uses of time and resources.* Washington, DC: American Psychological Association.

Committee on Managed Care of the American Psychiatric Association. (1983). *Utilization management: A handbook for psychiatrists.* Washington, DC: American Psychiatric Press.

Fitzpatrick, R. J., & Feldman, J. L. (Eds.). (1992). *Managed mental health care: Administrative and clinical issues.* Washington, DC: American Psychiatric Press.

Goodman, M., Brown, J., & Deitz, P. (1992). *Managing managed care.* Washington, DC: American Psychiatric Press.

Lowman, R. L. (Ed.). (1991). Special section on managed mental health care. *Professional Psychology: Research and Practice, 22*, 5–59.

Sharfstein, S., & Beigel, A. (Eds.). (1985). *The new economics and psychiatric care.* Washington, DC: American Psychiatric Press.

1

Current Mental Health Care Environments: Why Managed Care Is Necessary

Anthony Broskowski

This book is a testament to the fact that *managed care* is beginning to affect the practice of professional psychologists, and more important, that this trend is likely to continue. To practice effectively within such an environment, psychologists need to understand the forces promoting the growth of managed care and the ways they stand to be affected by and potentially to benefit from this major shift in the way mental health and substance abuse treatment services will be delivered in the future (Bloom, 1990). Although professional psychologists have not been primarily responsible for creating the cost trends that have stimulated managed care in mental health, they, like all other professionals, will be affected. It will not suffice to proclaim professional innocence, although professional sophistication on the issues may have some positive effects.

This chapter has four major purposes: (a) to review national trends in general health care costs and in health service delivery systems reacting to these cost trends; (b) to review comparable trends in mental health, drug, and alcohol treatment costs and service delivery systems that echo those in the general health system; (c) to make the case that managed care in the mental health industry arises as a marketplace response to concerns for service, cost, quality, and accessibility on the part of employers and insurers; and (d) to describe a general framework for understanding the structure of managed mental health care, while pointing to opportunities for psychologists who have cost-effective services to offer in a cost- and quality-competitive market.

National Health Care Costs

Trends in mental health can be viewed as an echo of trends occurring in the broader field of general health. Of these, the rising costs of treatment, even after accounting for general inflation, have been the dominant concern among

Reprinted from *Professional Psychology: Research and Practice, 22,* 6–14. (1991). Copyright 1991 by the American Psychological Association.

national policymakers and those sectors of the economy that end up paying the bill for treatment. In fact, the rising costs of care have been the primary factor motivating most of the other major changes taking place in the way services are financed, organized, and delivered.

In 1965, when Medicare and Medicaid were enacted, health expenditures of $39 billion represented only 6% of the gross national product (GNP). Per capita spending on health in 1965 was $181 (Sharfstein & Beigel, 1984). As recently as 1981 health care costs represented only 9.8% of the GNP (National Center for Health Statistics, 1982). By 1987, these costs were 11.1% of GNP. In 1990 they were expected to be between 11.3% and 12.5% of GNP, reaching 15% of GNP during the 1990s (Califano, 1986). Not only are health care costs increasing as a relative share of the GNP, but they are increasing at a relatively faster rate than are other categories of spending. Federal government expenditures on health grew 20% from 1987 to 1989, faster than Social Security increases (12.4%), military spending (5.7%), and interest on the national debt (17.8%; Freundenheim, 1988). Throughout the 1980s the rate of growth in health care spending exceeded the rate of inflation, as measured by the consumer price index (CPI; Berman, 1987). In 1987 Americans spent $500 billion on health care, up 9.6% over 1986, when inflation was only 4.4%. Whereas inflation has been running between 3% and 4%, the medical price index (MPI) has been running between 7% and 8% (Berman, 1987).

It is not just government spending on Medicaid, Medicare, and Civilian Health and Medical Programs of the Uniformed Services (CHAMPUS) populations that has fueled this phenomenon. Health care costs in 1984 represented 34% of corporate America's pretax profits (Califano, 1986). Lee Iacocca (Iacocca & Novak, 1984) credited health cost containment for some of Chrysler Corporation's successful turnaround. Iacocca wrote, "Blue Cross/Blue Shield had already become our largest supplier" (p. 306). Health care benefits were costing Chrysler $600 million annually, or $600 of the cost of producing a single car, and 7% of its sticker price. General Motors, the nation's largest employer, spent $2.9 billion on employee health benefits in 1987. American Telephone and Telegraph (AT&T) spent $1 billion (Freudenheim, 1988).

Although these large enterprises may appear to represent special circumstances, the pattern is consistent across small and medium companies as well. In its most recent annual survey of the health benefit costs of American employers (a representative sample of more than 1,600 large, medium, and small companies across 40 specific industries and representing over 10 million employees), Foster-Higgins (1989) highlighted significant trends in cost and employers' reactions to containing costs.

1. In 1984 the average per-employee cost for health care, including both employer's and employee's share, was $1,645; in 1985, it was $1,724; in 1986, it was $1,857; in 1987, it was $1,985; and in 1988 it rose steeply to $2,354, representing an increase of 18.6%.

2. The increase was experienced almost universally, with 88% of all respondents reporting an increase over 1987 costs.

3. There were only small variations in average costs due to geographical area ($2,000 to $2,500) and moderate variations based on type of industry

(more than \$3,000 in energy–petroleum, less than \$2,000 in retail–wholesale trades). Employers with over 40,000 employees had an average slightly above \$2,500, and those with fewer than 500 employees experienced an average of \$2,500.

Such relatively high costs for health care might not be of any concern if there were some visible return on the investment. But the unabated rate of increases, coupled with other economic indicators such as low productivity, has led some analysts to speculate that health care costs are a major threat to our country's ability to remain competitive in a world economy. Other modern nations generally spend far less per capita on health care, yet enjoy higher measures of population health, such as lower rates of child mortality and morbidity (Rice, 1988). For example, Japan spends only 6.7% of its GNP on health care, or \$500 per person, with no noted sacrifice (Califano, 1986).

Reasons for the Increase in Health Care Costs

To appreciate the range of strategies being used to contain health care costs, it is helpful to understand the general factors underlying the cost structure of health care:

$$Total\ Costs\ =\ (Unit\ Price)\ \times\ (Units\ Used).$$

Thus, the increase in health care costs can be traced to two general sets of factors: increasing prices charged for health services, and increasing health care utilization. For example, the National Center for Health Statistics estimates that increases in service utilization accounted for one third of the health care cost increases between 1965 and 1980, leaving two thirds driven by price increases (VandenBos, 1983). This chapter first examines the factors promoting price increases.

Since the end of World War II, hospital-based care has been the dominant contributor to rising health costs (Fox, 1984). Prior to 1983, hospitals were paid for care on the basis of a cost reimbursement. The hospital simply added on to its direct service costs whatever markup it chose for overhead and, where applicable, its profit. This payment philosophy finally ended in 1983, when the federal government introduced reimbursements for Medicare patients based on a prospectively fixed price, pegged to diagnostically related groupings (DRGs). Historically, insurance companies absorbed increases in hospital charges and passed them along to the employer in the form of higher insurance premiums. Although some insurance companies began using *usual and customary rates* (UCRs) as guidelines, these normative UCRs crept higher and higher as additional costs were incurred. Employees were buffered from cost increases by increasingly generous insurance plans. Direct payments by individuals accounted for only 25% of personal health care expenditures in 1987 (Health Care Finance Administration, 1988, cited in Group Health Association of America, 1990). Tax laws gave employers an incentive to increase benefits through tax-deductible health insurance rather than real cash wage and salary increases.

Consequently, hospitals had little incentive to operate efficiently and be cost-competitive. Federal health legislation also gave hospitals incentives to purchase new equipment, hire additional staff, and build additional space (Stokes & Rosala, 1978). Much of this expansion in capital equipment and buildings was financed by borrowing. Bankers happily lent money knowing that the hospitals could readily pass on the interest costs to their payers. Currently, hospitals are highly leveraged by debt, with debt-to-asset ratios as high as 80%. Thus, cost-plus payment for health care helps to stimulate cost-increasing behaviors on the part of care providers.

Insurance benefit plans created incentives for unnecessary hospital utilization by offering higher coverage for hospital-based care than for outpatient care. When outpatient costs were initially low, such copayment differentials did not necessarily promote hospitalization, but as outpatient charges rose, copayment requirements prompted physicians to encourage their patients to be treated in hospitals. Furthermore, physicians found a hospital-based practice to be increasingly convenient, remunerative, and conservative from the perspective of patient safety. Hospitals had no incentive to discourage inappropriate utilization. In fact, competition among hospitals was based not on price, but on their respective ability to attract the best admitting staff, often through perks and privileges, which contribute to further expenses then passed on to insurance companies and employers.

Other factors contributing to the current cost problems include demographics (specifically the age and health status of the population) and our changing societal perceptions on rights to health care.

The post-World War II baby boom is currently entering middle age, a time when use of health services increases as compared with youth. Along with age and an increasing use of medical service comes a profound shift in the type of health care needed and provided—from acute care for time-limited diseases or accidents to long-term care for chronic diseases and functional disabilities. Such forms of illness and their treatment require a greater expenditure for additional supportive services.

Another demographic fact has been the shift in our societal expectations regarding health care. Postwar research in such acute-care technologies as pharmaceuticals and surgery has created rising expectations of what health care can accomplish regardless of cost. Although such advances are laudable, they have been so well publicized by the mass media that the average citizen without training in economics or statistics has come to expect a cure for almost every common medical condition.

Paralleling the rise of informal expectations has been a growth in the legalization of expectations, through laws, regulations, and community standards of care. As more new types of medical care became hospital based, the standards for hospital care were expanded to cover them. Accreditation systems were also expanded to improve the quality of care. New biomedical technologies, funded through expanded research, were readily purchased by hospitals funded by cost-plus reimbursement. The new technologies tended to raise the legal standards of care and the expectations that all illnesses could be cured.

Increasing expectations, coupled with citizens' increasing sensitivity to their legal rights, raised the legal profession's interest in medical malpractice. To defend themselves against potential lawsuits, hospitals and doctors have had to incur even greater costs in equipment, testing, or additional treatments, just to meet the increasing standards of care of the community.

Technology continues to drive the costs of acute care. For example, immunosuppression research will further stimulate organ transplant capability. And although society applauds such increases in knowledge, their immediate and widespread application serves to raise expectations and the costs of providing such high-technology care. It is particularly perverse that the resources for such high-cost care are being spent on a very small number of patients, whose own lifestyles may have contributed to their medical conditions (Zook & Moore, 1980), while less expensive preventative care, such as adequate nutrition for young children, or prenatal care for young mothers, is not adequately financed on a comparable basis.

The lifestyles of many Americans, particularly those now entering their middle age, also affect health costs more generally. Smoking, overeating, poor nutrition, and stress-related behavior patterns have clearly added to increased health care use. But the skewed nature of the distribution among health care users is often not understood. Typically, there are a relatively few heavy hitters who strongly contribute to overall levels of use and cost. Zook and Moore (1980), for example, studied a random sample of 2,238 hospital records from 42,880 discharges among six different hospitals in Boston. They found that 13% of the high-cost users consumed as many resources as the other 87%. Extrapolating from the fact that 1 out of every 10 persons in the United States enters a hospital each year, the authors observe that "as few as 1.3% of the population consumes over half the hospital resources used in any given year" (p. 1001).

Furthermore, psychologists should be interested to know that the additional resource consumption was directly related to longer lengths of stay or higher readmission rates for the same episode of illness, and that approximately one half of these heavy users had illnesses related to their lifestyles, such as alcoholism, smoking, obesity, poor diet, or lack of behavioral compliance following their initial medical treatment.

Managed-Care Strategies Being Used to Contain Health Care Costs

By the mid 1970s, alarmed by health care costs, and understanding of some of the factors promoting its increase, the federal government, insurers, and employers began implementing a variety of mechanisms to contain cost increases (Herzlinger & Calkins, 1986). As with other major problems in American industry, it was decided that health care needed to be better managed. That meant focusing on utilization and unit price. For example, in 1983 the federal government introduced prospective payment for Medicare patients on the basis of DRGs. Instead of payment as a fee for service or as a premium pegged to a fixed amount per person at risk (capitation), this system pegs a fixed amount per type of disease or disorder.

Managed care has taken on a number of different meanings. To some it means any form of peer review to limit utilization, whereas others interpret it to mean active case management of a patient's treatment to coordinate and assure continuity of care. In fact, these are only two of the many mechanisms used in managed-care systems. Although some of these mechanisms can be used in isolation, when several are organized in a coherent fashion, they constitute one of various types of managed-care systems, most notably health maintenance organizations (HMOs) and preferred provider organizations (PPOs).

In addition, there now exists a new breed of organization best described as a *case management organization* (CMO). CMOs will combine one or more of the various mechanisms into a service product to be sold to insurers and employers. This product is neither an HMO nor a PPO, although elements of prepayment, capitation, or discounted provider networks may be used. Some CMOs offer generic medical and surgical case management, and others specialize in specific disorders such as psychiatric and substance abuse or work-related disabilities.

The primary mechanisms currently being used to reduce utilization include (a) pretreatment authorization, (b) concurrent utilization review, (c) benefit plans designed to provide financial incentives or constraints for receiving care from efficient providers, and (d) increasing requirements for greater employee–user cost sharing.

The primary mechanisms being used to control price include (a) capitated payments for a defined group of beneficiaries, (b) negotiated fee-for-service payments to preferred providers selected for quality and efficiency, (c) prospective fixed payments for DRGs, (d) claims review, and (e) insurance coverage extended to cover less expensive but equally effective treatment alternatives (Foster-Higgins, 1989). The application of these mechanisms to psychiatric disorders and their implications for mental health service organizations are further reviewed in Broskowski and Marks (1990).

Redistributing the Risks for Utilization and Costs

Another way to look at insurance and managed-care systems is to analyze the ways they attempt to redistribute the risks of utilization and the cost of treatment among (a) the employee or potential at-risk user; (b) the patient or actual user; (c) the provider of care; (d) the employer; and (e) the insurer or managed-care organization. Historically, totally private, self-pay, fee-for-service health care put only the patient–user at risk for utilization and costs. In recent decades the employer assumed responsibility but paid premiums to an insurance company to assume all or most of the risks of variability in utilization and treatment prices. Sometimes insurance premiums are paid in part by the employees, who thereby assume some of the risks whether or not they ever use medical services. Copayments and deductibles further allocate utilization and price risks to those who actually use services. In some plans there is some maximum limit placed on the users' financial responsibility through *stop-loss* provisions.

In managed care the provider is asked to assume some risks or to contribute to the total cost of care by either (a) agreeing to provide services for a discounted fee or (b) agreeing to provide all care for a prepaid per capita rate. Giving fee-for-service discounts puts the provider at risk for cost controls and some service utilization variability depending upon the unit of service being negotiated, as when a hospital offers an all-inclusive discount per diem rate. Capitation systems put the provider at risk for variable rates of use among all potential users as well as the amount of actual use by each patient.

The managed-care company, which may be an insurance company, HMO, PPO, or CMO, may assume total or partial risks by indemnifying the employer for all or some of the costs of care. When it assumes all of the financial risks, as in the case of true indemnity insurers, it will retain any savings as profits. It may assume only some of the total risks by having the fees it is paid for its services tied to the level of savings achieved, or it may assume limited responsibility for a percentage of the treatment costs that exceeded an agreed target level. In some cases the managed-care entity may get a share of savings or a performance bonus. Some managed-care systems, such as closed-panel HMOs, combine the provider's risks with the insurer's risk through direct employment of the service provider.

Cost savings in managed-care systems can be achieved through at least three mechanisms: (a) the diversion of patients from inpatient treatment to less restrictive but equally effective outpatient care, such as day–evening substance abuse programs as alternatives to 28-day inpatient stays (Miller & Hester, 1986; Hayashida et al., 1989) or partial hospital programs (Sharfstein, 1985); (b) the reduction of unnecessarily long hospital stays; and (c) price discounts offered by preferred providers who in turn receive an increased volume of patient referrals. In addition, benefit plans may provide incentives for employees to seek early telephonic assessment and triage services, followed by ongoing case management of all care, whether by preferred (i.e., contracted) or nonpreferred providers, and for all levels of treatment. Such programs may also include claims preprocessing to compare the number and type of services authorized by the clinical case manager with the provider's billed charges.

Thus, managed care can refer to a variety of mechanisms designed to control utilization or costs. These mechanisms range from externally imposed monitoring and control systems put in place before, during, or after the point of service or claims payment to economic incentives or risk distribution systems intended to establish self-monitored efficiency and effectiveness in treatment-seeking or treatment-giving behaviors.

Health Care Providers' Responses to Managed Care

The cost-containment mechanisms used by payers also stimulated reactions in the provider systems, many of which can be subsumed under the general rubric of *proprietary health care*. Although most hospitals after World War II were either owned by the government or by not-for-profit charitable or religious organizations, in the 1970s there was an increase of private, for-profit hospitals, many of which became investor owned. Health care became a big industry with potential profits, and it attracted many investors and entrepreneurs.

As health care technology, administration, and financing became increasingly complex, new organizational forms were created to deal with the complexity (Broskowski, 1987). Strategies used in other industries were adopted by the health care industry. Vertical integration increased as hospitals invested in alternative levels of treatment, including outpatient and home health care. Joint ventures, mergers, and consolidations among hospital and medical group practices began to occur. Multiple hospitals were organized as chains, many of which were financed through stock ownership.

Horizontal integration also occurred, as formally separate and distinct sectors—employers, insurance companies, and hospitals—began to blur their former boundaries. Hospital chains formed joint ventures with insurance companies to improve market share and to control costs. Hospital supply companies and hospitals formed joint ventures.

Most large employers shifted to self-funded insurance, some to save the profits being made by their former insurance companies, others to avoid the mandated insurance benefits lobbied into state insurance laws by self-interested provider organizations. In its national survey of 1,633 employers, Foster-Higgins (1989) reported that 65% of employers with more than 1,000 employees shifted to self-funded insurance, compared with only 41% of those with fewer than 1,000 employees. Overall, 48% were self-funded. These self-insured employers' benefit plans are governed by the federal Employee Retirement Income Security Act of 1974 (ERISA) and are exempt from most state insurance requirements. The insurance companies now serving these self-insured employers act only as administrators of claims payment and, in many cases, provide the various managed-care services of utilization review and case management.

At the same time that payers (government and private employers) were seeking to control utilization and price, the supply of institutional and private practice providers continued to increase. Most certificate-of-need and health-planning legislation failed to stem the multiplication of hospital beds in the face of the attractive profits to be made. Professional schools continued to produce an oversupply of specialists, and the concentration of hospitals and related health resources in urban communities led to a serious maldistribution of the available resources. The supply–demand–cost cycle continues when the relative oversupply of providers, seeking a reduced set of insured patients, stimulates further competitive behaviors, such as cutting prices or stimulating demand through advertising. Providers modify their practice patterns, and patients modify their expectations of free choice and unlimited utilization. In brief, health care is now responding to some basic laws of economics, including responsiveness to price and quality differentials among providers.

Cost Considerations in Mental Health and Substance Abuse Care

Although less well documented, the costs of treating alcohol, drug abuse, and mental health (ADM) problems has been steadily increasing, and doing so at a relatively faster rate than have the costs of treating other insured conditions (Frank & Kamlet, 1985). In a recent survey by the Employee Benefit Information Center (TPF&C, 1989), 62% of the responding companies reported experiencing a greater proportional increase in ADM costs than in other medical costs. Twenty percent experienced increases in the range of 10% to 19%, and another one fifth reported increases in the range of 20% to 29%. In the Foster-Higgins (1989) survey respondents reported a 27% increase in ADM costs, from an average of $163 per employee to more than $207. In that sample of over 1,600 employers, ADM expenditures accounted for 9.6% of total medical plan costs. Many employers who have chosen to use case management systems have average ADM costs exceeding $250, and in some cases more than $600, per employee.

Although cost-containment strategies for general medical care, primarily hospital-based care, have begun to pay off through reductions in length of stays and cost of episodes, (Teitelman, 1985), the costs for ADM treatment episodes have been increasing. Whereas ADM costs historically averaged as little as 2% to 5% of funds expended on insured medical care, they now represent 10% to 20% of such costs among many large, self-insured employers (Wallace, 1987). Many employers now report that ADM episodes are among the most expensive of all types of episodes for which they pay insurance claims. A typical 28-day stay for alcohol or drug treatment in 1990 could easily cost more than $15,000 when all room and board, ancillary, and professional charges were included. John Erb of Foster-Higgins estimated that psychiatric and substance abuse costs increased in 1989 by more than 50% (Schiffman, 1989).

Treatment costs for ADM are also distributed unevenly across treatment settings and users. Depending on the nature of the benefit, 65% to 80% of costs are likely to be incurred in inpatient and residential settings, although only 10% to 20% of all users use such care. Among inpatient users it is not unusual to find less than 50% of the admissions accounting for 80% of the total inpatient costs. Regarding outpatient treatment, the National Medical Care Utilization and Expenditure Survey indicated that 44% of outpatient users made 4 or fewer visits and accounted for only 6.7% of total expenditures, whereas 16.2% of outpatients made more than 24 visits and accounted for 57.4% of costs (Taube, Kessler, & Feuerberg, 1984).

The reasons for the increasing costs in ADM treatment are similar to those applying to general health care. Although there have been few costly high technologies introduced into the ADM field, utilization has dramatically increased, particularly in private psychiatric and general medical hospitals (Kiesler & Sibulkin, 1984, 1987). Many general hospitals opened psychiatric units because charges for such disorders were exempted from the Medicare DRG payment system. Not only were ADM services reimbursed on a fee-for-service basis, but psychiatric beds are less expensive to operate than are medical beds, and they can produce a higher margin of return on investment. Many of the vacant beds resulting from reduced medical admissions and lengths of stay for Medicare and private patients were profitably converted to psychiatric or substance abuse units.

The number of private psychiatric hospitals in the United States increased from 180 to 250 between 1970 and 1985, and the number of psychiatric beds owned and operated by private hospital chains increased by about 15% in 1984 (Sullivan, Flynn, & Lewin, 1987). Bickman and Dokecki (1989), in an excellent summary of cyclical trends affecting the balance of private and public responsibilities for mental health services, described the increase in concentration of ownership of psychiatric hospitals by private chains. Currently, only four corporations own 59% of all private for-profit hospitals.

Some ADM utilization increase is because a lot of mental illness went unrecognized and untreated in previous decades. If treated, it was frequently uninsured. If insured and treated, it often went unclaimed by the employee–patient because of the fear of stigma. If a claim was submitted, the level of coverage, and hence the employer's share of the costs, were relatively low.

Now the cost of ADM care is increasing for all major employers, for several reasons: (a) There is less stigma against mental illness and its treatment in the current generation of employed citizens, (b) there has been a real increase in the use of drugs and alcohol across all age groups in the population, (c) popular culture has popularized many forms of psychotherapy and personal growth, and (d) government support for community-based mental health treatment and financial support for the training and education of mental health professionals have promoted an increase in the availability of providers (Pepe & Wu, 1988). With an increased supply of providers comes increased utilization, and a relative excess in the supply of providers increases competition for the finite number of insured patients. Competition leads providers to further encourage utilization through a variety of practice-building behaviors, including advertising. Sometimes these practices may have helped those who might not otherwise have sought care. In many other cases, these practices have encouraged people to seek a form of care that is much more expensive than necessary but less effective.

Paralleling the trends in health services delivery systems is a vertical integration of ADM treatment resources, manifest in such concepts as *treatment continuum* and *continuity of services*. This trend is especially dominant for such expensive-to-treat, at-risk populations as chronically mentally ill adults and seriously disturbed adolescents (Behar, Macbeth, & Holland, 1993). Certainly the growth of private ADM hospital chains also attests to increasing integration of resources. These hospitals, as well as private practice groups, are also now responding to the economic realities of managed care by establishing such inpatient alternatives as day and evening partial hospital programs and outpatient clinics. Such organizational trends in mental health are likely to continue and have significant implications for how mental health professionals organize and manage themselves and their traditionally private practices (Broskowski, 1987). Finally, there continues to be great interest in the quality and cost-effectiveness gains to be realized by integrating mental health services more effectively into the broader delivery of primary and selected specialty (e.g., pediatrics) medical services (Bloom, 1990; Broskowski, 1982; Broskowski, Marks, & Budman, 1981).

The range of reactions among mental health providers has not been very different from that observed among general medical providers at the onset of managed care. At one extreme is denial or rage and resistance, characterized by outright refusal to cooperate with utilization review, efforts to introduce legislation or regulations to prevent or inhibit managed care, and publications about the dire results for the patients that can be expected to stem from managed care (Melnick & Lyter, 1987). It is an unusual article that does not refer to the effects managed care is having on the autonomy or the profitability of private facilities or private practices (Ludwigsen & Enright, 1988). Other providers become involved in appropriate efforts to create proper standards to guard against potential abuses. Still others begin to respond by modifying their practice patterns or developing better treatment alternatives.

Scope and Effectiveness of Managed Health and Alcohol, Drug Abuse, and Mental Health Care

One cannot examine the scope or effectiveness of managed care of ADM treatment independently of managed care of general health because the former is often done within the context of the latter. Specifically, as more health care is affected by mechanisms of managed care, employers are simply extending these mechanisms to their ADM insurance coverage.

The first conclusion is that the use of managed-care systems in health and mental health is increasing. Foster-Higgins (1989) reported that 68% of its employer respondents required precertification of elective hospital admissions, with 73% of large employers (i.e., with more than 1,000 employees) doing so. Concurrent review of hospital care is required by 61% of large employers and 37% of smaller ones. Most cover second opinions for surgery and many require it. For those respondents who were able to estimate savings, most reported that utilization review alone saved them 5% to 6% of total costs. There has also been a steady growth in HMO enrollments since they were first offered by employers. In recent years, however, there has been a leveling off at around 35% of the insured workforce, and Foster-Higgins reported (1989) that some employers are beginning to reduce the number of HMOs they offer to employees. Employers are also divided in their opinions about the savings they achieve through HMO enrollments. Many report increases in their indemnity insurance plans as the healthy employees elect HMO membership, leaving the higher risk patients in the indemnity plan. Melnick, Zwanziger, and Verity-Guerra (1989) also reported initial growth and now a leveling of HMO plans nationally, with 165 plans and 6.3 million subscribers in 1977, growing to 662 plans with 28.6 million subscribers. The financial failures among HMOs in recent years have made employers wary of this option for their employees.

The percentage of employers offering PPOs continues to increase, especially among large employers (Foster-Higgins, 1989). PPOs are arrangements by which financial or other incentives are offered to covered individuals who utilize preselected care providers. The employer's incentive is reduced costs through provider discounts, and the provider is attracted to the prospect of a broadened referral base. Sixty percent of employers using PPOs agreed that they were effective in reducing costs, with savings ranging as high as 10%

with an average of 3.3%. Reviewing the growth of selective contracting of hospitals, beginning in California in 1982, Melnick et al. (1989) reported national increases in PPO growth, from 73 PPO plans in 1983 to 575 in 1988. Enrollment levels were unknown in 1983, but were 1.3 million in 1984 and grew to 35 million by 1988, comprising 16.56% of the non-Medicare population. Employers are finding that their health care costs can be controlled, and in some cases reduced below their currently high levels (Alt, 1988; Fine, 1988).

Effectiveness of Managed Care

Employers are as interested in evaluating their managed-care vendors as they are in having these vendors monitor the direct service providers (Milstein, Oehm, & Alpert, 1987). Consequently, there have been numerous studies and surveys on managed-care effectiveness (Curtiss, 1989), with most reporting positive results using cost-saving criteria. For example, Feldstein, Wickizer, and Wheeler (1988) analyzed insurance claims over 2 years on 222 groups of employees and dependents covered by a large insurance carrier with a compulsory utilization review (UR) program. They reported that, after controlling for employee characteristics, market factors, and benefit plan features, UR reduced admissions by 12.3%, inpatient days by 8.0%, hospital expenditures by 11.9%, and total medical expenditures by 8.3%, with a savings-to-cost ratio of approximately 8 to 1.

Melnick et al. (1989) noted that selective contracting (i.e., PPOs) in California has dramatically reduced such indicators as cost per admission and cost per day among hospitals, which before 1982 exceeded national averages but after the introduction of the PPO were below them. They also reported that in 1974 the percentages of per capita spending on hospital services in California and the nation were the same, 2.71%, but had increased in California from 1974 to 1982, peaking at 3.8%, whereas the national average peaked at 3.96%. In 1983, prospective payment systems were introduced, and this index began to decline both nationally and in California. By 1986 it was 3.56% for California and 4.03% nationally.

Improvements in the quality of care (an often-neglected managed-care variable) have been harder to demonstrate. However, opponents of managed care have found it equally difficult to demonstrate any loss of quality. Although definitive studies of differential levels in patient outcomes are lacking, there is documented evidence that managed care has reduced the amount of inappropriate care being rendered (Siu et al., 1986) and has eliminated significant levels of fraudulent and abusive practices among providers (Califano, 1986).

Surveys of beneficiary satisfaction with managed care reflect increasing acceptance. Alvine (1989), reporting on a recent survey by the Metropolitan Life Insurance Company of 50 union leaders and 50 corporate executives that compared their opinions on managed care and traditional health insurance, indicated that 46% of union leaders said quality had not changed, 28% thought it had improved, 13% thought it had become worse, and 13% had formed no opinion. The respective figures for corporate leaders were 63%, 28%, 5%, and 4%.

Anderson (1989) compared three types of UR organizations in their relative effectiveness in controlling ADM average lengths of stay (ALOS) and the quality of patient care provided, as rated by board-certified psychiatrists examining the full medical records of the reviewed cases. The three types of UR organizations were (a) psychiatric UR firms using a specialty PPO, (b) specialized UR only, and (c) nonspecialized UR only. The first group had an ALOS of 9 days, the second had an ALOS of 16 days, and the third had an ALOS of 18.2 days. The possible quality-of-care ratings for each case were *poor*, *acceptable*, and *good*. There were few differences between the three types of UR firms in the percentage of cases rated poor (21%, 16%, 31%), acceptable (53%, 49%, 44%), or good (26%, 34%, 25%).

Burton, Hoy, Bonin, and Gladstone (1989) describe a before-and-after comparison of a program of prevention and early intervention, hospital UR, and the services of a consulting psychiatrist, on the cost, utilization, and rated quality of psychiatric hospitalization for 12,500 insured lives. There were 76 annual admissions before the program, and 76 during the 12 months of the program, but inpatient days were reduced by 43%, and costs were reduced by 32%. A major reduction in admission rates occurred for the diagnostic category of anxiety (12 vs. 1). The authors claimed that reviews of preprogram medical charts revealed deterioration in some patients due to prolonged stays, compared with improved quality for misdiagnosed cases due to the intervention of the consulting psychiatrist during the program.

These findings may prompt clinicians to question the impact of such programs on the patients' care. This legitimate concern is increasingly being addressed by managed-care firms' analyses of clinical outcomes. Although such clinical-outcome results are not yet systematically available, it is clear that managed care does extend the range of treatments available to patients when case managers are given the authority to override the narrow restrictions of written benefit plans and to certify a range of alternative treatments. For example, a hospitalized adolescent's discharge plan and continuity of care may be enhanced by the case manager's ability to authorize innovative home-based, school-based, and office-based alternative services that, in a nonmanaged situation, would not be covered by the benefit plan, (Behar et al., 1993). The accumulating evidence suggests that there are many cost-effective substitutes and complements to traditional inpatient treatment (Goldstein & Horgan, 1988). Moreover, Brightbill (1988) reported that, in some cases of managed care, admissions rates may actually increase while days per 1,000 lives are reduced and overall costs are reduced through the providers' price discounts.

It is not uncommon to observe an increase in the number of outpatient users and an increase in the average number of outpatient visits per episode at the same time that unnecessary inpatient care is reduced. In some cases the employer's costs of managed ADM outpatient care exceed the costs for ADM inpatient care. To the extent that more employees are using their ADM benefits and experiencing greater continuity of treatment within and across more appropriate types of treatment, it could be said that managed care has improved quality by improving access to the most qualified providers. And through encouraging continuity, managed care has improved the potential of forestalling more serious levels of disability and maintaining care over the long run.

Contrary to the beliefs of many providers, employers' interests in managed care are not based exclusively on economic factors. They are also concerned with the quality of care and are aware that most employees cannot adequately determine the type of the care they need. Furthermore, analysts understand that cost and quality are related in several ways (Mechanic, 1985; Steffen, 1988). Poor quality of care usually leads to additional care, at added cost, for the same problems. Fragmented care may be of lower quality, because the synergistic effects of a coordinated system of care are not present. By managing care, employers hope to enhance clinical effectiveness by encouraging more coordinated, appropriate care. This emphasis allows for a shift in utilization patterns to less restrictive settings, and for the possibility of even more successful outcomes.

Implications for the Practice of Psychology

This chapter has been a broad review of the cost rationale for managed care, and as such does not allow a detailed review of the opportunities that managed care offers for psychologists. However, there is a growing literature on managed care and the alternative ways it is organized and made available in the marketplace. Psychologists seeking to grow within the managed-care industry would be well advised to read more about how it can operate within and across different employers, insurers, and providers. For an excellent summary of these trends and their implications for psychologists, see Kiesler and Morton's (1988) article, "Psychology and Public Policy in the 'Health Care Revolution.'" The clues for psychologists in managed care are embedded in such concepts as supply and demand, cost-effectiveness, competition, distribution, continuity, and cost containment. Although these are fairly new terms and concepts for clinical services, they are not necessarily incompatible with such traditional values as autonomy, quality, free choice, confidentiality, and easy access to needed services.

Because psychologists historically have not been associated with inpatient care, their future opportunities are embedded in their ability to design cost-effective alternatives, particularly modalities that deliver the care within the patient's natural settings, such as the home or school. Psychologists interested in direct clinical services can focus their efforts in several specific areas. For example, office-based psychologists should begin to develop and emphasize their skills in brief planned therapy (Budman & Gurman, 1988; MacKenzie, 1988) and lower cost behavioral approaches to common disorders and disabilities. Others can consider providing work-site or in-home services. In some cases managed-care companies will pay a premium fee for on-call services or scheduled visits in the home. Insurers and managed-care firms are also contracting with clinicians to serve as their direct agents on a capitated or fee-for-service basis to conduct on-site, face-to-face assessments of hospital patients for whom they are seeking a second opinion about the necessity of hospitalization, or seeking a better developed discharge plan.

Because of cost controls, providers and patients will continue to experience an erosion of free choice and unlimited services, but quality will continue to be a major concern because managed care must come to grips with the cost of poor quality. The debate among providers, employers, and payers will center around the best operational definitions of quality. But the burden of proof is also shifting to the provider. Traditional inpatient services, regardless of their acceptance among professionals, will not necessarily be accepted as quality by others. Conversely, new types of outpatient services, never before reimbursable, are now in an excellent position to demonstrate their relative cost-effectiveness. Psychologists trained to understand and value research should be at an advantage in a marketplace concerned with financial and clinical accountability. To the extent that they are willing and able to demonstrate more cost-effective treatments, psychologists are in a good position to increase their market share relative to other disciplines (Broskowski, 1989). Although the disciplines may compete or try to prevent competition through statutory and regulatory barriers to entry into the marketplace, the forces of economics are likely to outlast any short-term disciplinary rivalries and their associated tactics. This is not to imply that psychologists do not have to defend their hard-earned professional privileges and seek equity wherever appropriate. But the competition is truly in the managed-care marketplace, where cost and outcomes are being examined and evaluated continuously.

Beyond traditional clinical practice, psychologists can show leadership in organizing and managing comprehensive, multidisciplinary group practices that expand the range of available services by incorporating effective alternatives to more expensive care, such as partial hospital programs, and integrated family services, including in-home crisis intervention, therapeutic foster families, and short-term group homes for children who truly need to be removed from their natural homes. Again, space limits a full review of the organizational, managerial, and financial requirements for such ventures, but they are clearly viable strategies for well-balanced groups of professionals with adequate managerial sophistication within their group.

Another strategy is to organize selected providers into their own PPO, UR, or case-management organization, taking some of the risks for overutilization and costs through negotiated contracts with employers or insurers. Many large insurers cannot efficiently provide well-focused ADM utilization review or case-management services to smaller employers or large employers with employees in small communities. In organizing and marketing such services, however, one needs to be very careful in analyzing the cost structures of the particular clinical or case-management services to be offered and the utilization patterns among the groups of employees for which services will be offered. This caution is particularly important for those considering discounted clinical service fees, or the assumption of partial risks or cost-savings performance contracts on a capitated basis (Broskowski & Marks, 1990). It is often easy to begin offering utilization review or case management on a case-by-case fee basis or for a percentage of treatment costs saved. There are also other issues that need to be addressed, such as avoiding incentive systems that represent a conflict of interest, carrying adequate malpractice coverage, and observing all applicable laws, regulations, and ethical guidelines.

Psychologists should also consider the expanded opportunities for employment as managers or consultants working within this managed-care industry. Large employers, insurance companies, the large benefit-management consulting firms, and the specialized managed-care companies are seeking help in controlling costs while maintaining quality. Psychologists whose training spans clinical and research domains can bring an excellent combination of skills to such firms, whose current workforces are predominantly staffed by medical professionals, psychiatrists, nurses, or clinical social workers.

As mental illness, drugs, and alcohol problems continue to grow as threats to the American economy, business and political leaders will look for solutions. I hope they will be able to turn to well-qualified psychologists as much as they now turn to their accountants and auditors. Psychologists must be prepared, however, to participate in these, or better, managed-care solutions, and not simply argue for more of the same private, uncontrolled, and often guild-oriented fee-for-service systems of the past.

References

Alt, S. (1988). Xerox spends money to save money on mental health care. *Contract Healthcare*, 39–40.

Alvine, R. (1989). Data watch: Labor issues for the 1990s. *Business & Health, 7*, 12.

Anderson, D. (1989). How effective is managed mental health care? *Business and Health, 7*, 34–35.

Behar, L., Macbeth, G., & Holland, J. (1993). Distribution of mental health services and their costs within a system of care for seriously emotionally disturbed and at risk children and adolescents. *Administration and Policy in Mental Health, 20*, 283–295.

Berman, K. (1987). Health insurance rates keep climbing. *Business Insurance, 21*, 1, 34.

Bickman, L., & Dokecki, P. (1989). Public and private responsibility for mental health services. *American Psychologist, 44*, 1138–1141.

Bloom, B. (1990). Managing mental health services: Some comments for the overdue debate in psychology. *Community Mental Health Journal, 26*, 107–124.

Brightbill, T. (1988, July). Mental health firms offer more care for less costs. *Contract Healthcare*, 9–11.

Broskowski, A. (1982). Linking mental health and health care systems. In H. C. Schulberg & M. Killilea (Eds.), *The modern practice of community mental health*. San Francisco, Jossey-Bass.

Broskowski, A. (1987). Goldfields and minefields: Changing management technologies and resources. *Administration in Mental Health, 14*, 153–171.

Broskowski, A. (1989). Challenges and opportunities for researchers in managed care systems. In P. Greenbaum, R. Friedman, A. Duchnowski, K. Kutash, & S. Silver (Eds.), *Children's mental health services and policies: Building a research base*. Tampa: University of South Florida, Florida Mental Health Institute.

Broskowski, A., & Marks, E. (1990). Managed mental health care. In T. Lentner & S. Cooper (Eds.), *Innovations in community mental health*. Sarasota, FL: Professional Resource Exchange.

Broskowski, A., Marks, E., & Budman, S. (Eds.). (1981). *Linking health and mental health: Coordinating care in the community*. Beverly Hills, CA: Sage.

Budman, S., & Gurman, A. (1988). *Theory and practice of brief therapy*. New York: Guilford Press.

Burton, W., Hoy, D., Bonin, R., & Gladstone, L. (1989). Quality and cost-effective management of mental health care. *Journal of Occupational Medicine, 31,* 363–366.

Califano, J. A., Jr. (1986). *America's health care revolution: Who lives? Who dies? Who pays?* New York: Random House.

Curtiss, F. (1989). How managed care works. *Personnel Journal, 68,* 38–53.

Feldstein, P., Wickizer, T., & Wheeler, J. (1988). Private cost containment: The effects of utilization review programs on health care use and expenditures. *New England Journal of Medicine, 318,* 1310–1314.

Fine, M. (1988). Managing mental health care greatly lowers costs. *Managed Care Outlook, 1,* 3–4.

Foster-Higgins. (1989). *Health care benefits survey, 1988*. Princeton, NJ: Author.

Fox, P. (1984). Plan design. In P. Fox, W. Goldbeck, & J. Spies (Eds.), *Health care cost management*. Ann Arbor, MI: Health Administration Press.

Frank, R., & Kamlet, M. (1985). Direct costs and expenditures for mental health care in the United States in 1980. *Hospital and Community Psychiatry, 36,* 165–168.

Freudenheim, M. (1988, November 19). U.S. health care spending continues sharp rise. *The New York Times,* p. A1.

Goldstein, J., & Horgan, C. (1988). Inpatient and outpatient psychiatric services: Substitutes or complements? *Hospital and Community Psychiatry, 39,* 632–636.

Group Health Association of America. (1990). By the numbers. *GHAA News, 31,* 27.

Hayashida, M., Alterman, A., McLellan, T., O'Brien, C., Purtill, J., Volpicelli, J., Raphaelson, A., & Hall, C. (1989). Comparative effectiveness and costs of inpatient and outpatient detoxification of patients with mild-to-moderate alcohol withdrawal syndrome. *New England Journal of Medicine, 320,* 358–365.

Herzlinger, R., & Calkins, D. (1986). How companies tackle health care costs: Part III. *Harvard Business Review, 64,* 70–80.

Iacocca, L., & Novak, W. (1984). *Iacocca: An autobiography*. New York: Bantam Books.

Kiesler, C., & Morton, T. (1988). Psychology and public policy in the "health care revolution." *American Psychologist, 43,* 993–1003.

Kiesler, C., & Sibulkin, A. (1984). Episodic rate of mental hospitalization: Stable or increasing? *American Journal of Psychiatry, 141,* 44–48.

Kiesler, C., & Sibulkin, A. (1987). *Mental hospitalization: Myths and facts about a national crisis*. Newbury Park, CA: Sage.

Ludwigsen, K., & Enright, M. (1988). The health care revolution: Implications for psychology and hospital practice. *Psychotherapy, 25,* 424–428.

MacKenzie, K. (1988). Recent developments in brief psychotherapy. *Hospital and Community Psychiatry, 39,* 742–752.

Mechanic, D. (1985). Cost containment and the quality of medical care: Rationing strategies in an era of constrained resources. *Milbank Memorial Fund Quarterly: Health and Society, 63,* 453–475.

Melnick, S., & Lyter, L. (1987). The negative impacts of increased concurrent review of psychiatric inpatient care. *Hospital and Community Psychiatry, 38,* 300–302.

Melnick, G., Zwanziger, J., & Verity-Guerra, A. (1989). The growth and effects of hospital selective contracting. *Health Care Management Review, 14,* 57–64.

Miller, W., & Hester, R. (1986). Inpatient alcoholism treatment: Who benefits? *American Psychologist, 41,* 794–805.

Milstein, A., Oehm, M., & Alpert, G. (1987). Gauging the performance of utilization review. *Business and Health, 4,* 10–12.

National Center for Health Statistics. (1982). *Health, United States* (DHHS Publication No. PHS 83-1232). Washington, DC: U.S. Government Printing Office.

Pepe, M., & Wu, J. (1988). The economics of mental health care. *Psychotherapy, 25,* 352–355.

Rice, D. (1988). Do we get full value for our health dollar? *Hospitals, 62,* 18.

Schiffman, J. (1989, November 10). Health costs. *The Wall Street Journal,* p. B1.

Sharfstein, S. (1985). Financial incentives for alternatives to hospital care. *Psychiatric Clinics of North America, 8,* 449–460.

Sharfstein, S., & Beigel, A. (1984). Less is more? Today's economics and its challenge to psychiatry. *American Journal of Psychiatry, 141*, 1403–1408.

Siu, A., Sonnenberg, F., Manning, W., Goldberg, G., Bloomfield, E., Newhouse, J., & Brook, R. (1986). Inappropriate use of hospitals in a randomized trial of health insurance plans. *The New England Journal of Medicine, 315*, 1259–1266.

Steffen, G. (1988). Quality medical care. *Journal of the American Medical Association, 260*, 56–61.

Stokes, L., & Rosala, J. (1978). *How business can improve health planning and regulation.* Washington, DC: National Chamber Foundation.

Sullivan, S., Flynn, T., & Lewin, M. (1987). The quest to manage mental health costs. *Business and Health, 4*, 24–28.

TPF&C. (1989). *Psychiatric and substance abuse cost survey.* Valhalla, NY: TPF&C Employee Benefits Information Center.

Taube, C., Kessler, L., & Feuerberg, M. (1984). Utilization and expenditures for ambulatory mental health care during 1980. *National medical care utilization and expenditure survey: Data report 5.* Washington, DC: U.S. Department of Health and Human Services.

Teitelman, R. (1985, June). No shrinkage for the shrinks. *Forbes,* p. 174.

VandenBos, G. (1983). Health financing, service utilization, and national policy: A conversation with Stan Jones. *American Psychologist, 38*, 948–955.

Wallace, C. (1987, July). Employers turning to managed care to control their psychiatric care costs. *Modern Healthcare,* pp. 82–84.

Zook, C., & Moore, F. (1980). High-cost users of medical care. *New England Journal of Medicine, 302*, 996–1002.

2

Managed Mental Health Care: A History of the Federal Policy Initiative

Patrick H. DeLeon,
Gary R. VandenBos,
and Elizabeth Q. Bulatao

The true beginning of the modern concept of *managed health care* is somewhat obscure. There are events in the early 1900s that could lead one to agree to a date like 1904 or 1906. With the Ross-Loos Clinic becoming operational in 1929, that year has a good claim. The Depression-era efforts of Kaiser Permanente became fully recognized in 1945, so that date stands out. The passage of the federal Health Maintenance Organization Act in 1973 can be viewed as a central date as well.

The lumbering and mining industries operating in the Pacific Northwest in the early 1900s provided the site of an early prepayment plan—that is, the provision of a set package of health care services by an identified provider for a preestablished fee. The Western Clinic, a fee-for-service partnership in Tacoma, Washington, is reported to be one of the first prepaid group practices. In 1906, two physicians contracted to provide medical care for lumber employees for 50¢ per individual per month. Physicians in private practice in Tacoma, in opposition to the prepaid concept, organized the Pierce County Medical Service Bureau and attempted to limit competition and became a predecessor of county medical societies (Bennett, 1988; Flinn, McMahon, & Collins, 1987).

The combination of prepayment schemes with group practice arrangements began in the 1920s. In the mid-1920s, a prepaid system for farmers in cooperatives in rural Oklahoma was initiated. In 1929, the Ross-Loos Medical Group contracted with the employees of the Los Angeles County Department of Water and Power and their families for a consumer-controlled comprehensive health care program.

The Kaiser Permanente Health Plan is another forerunner to the modern health maintenance organization (HMO). The Kaiser Permanente version of managed health care was born in the Mojave Desert of California during the

Reprinted from *Professional Psychology: Research and Practice, 22,* 15–25. (1991). Copyright 1991 by the American Psychological Association.

1930s. After receiving the contract to build the aqueduct from Boulder Dam (later renamed Hoover Dam) to Los Angeles, builder Henry J. Kaiser had difficulty recruiting and maintaining adequate construction crews in the desert. Workers were reluctant to move their families there, in large part because of the lack of medical care. Hearing of this problem, a young physician named Sidney Garfield offered to provide all of the facilities and services necessary for comprehensive health care for workers and their families at a cost of 5¢ per employee work hour. A unique feature of the plan was preventive—primarily against sunstroke and exhaustion, which are perils of the desert (Cummings & VandenBos, 1981).

In 1937, the Group Health Association (GHA) opened in Washington, DC, becoming the first HMO on the east coast. Group Health Association is a nonprofit membership corporation with, in 1989, about 150,000 members or covered individuals. The majority (55%) of its participants are commercial or corporate group employees; 40% are federal employees covered under the Federal Employees Health Benefits Plan (FEHBP); and about 5% are direct payers or individuals having personal coverage (J. Schlosser, GHA, personal communication, February 23, 1990).

At the end of World War II the Kaiser Permanente Health Plan went public and immediately flourished. Its early acceptance was obviously because the plan provided comprehensive treatment for all problems at low subscriber rates, without the exclusions, limitations, high out-of-pocket cost sharing, and other troublesome features common to other health plans at the time. Kaiser Permanente would later become a pioneer in the provision of comprehensive mental health care as an integral part of a total, prepaid health care delivery system (Cummings & VandenBos, 1981).

The HMO movement, from 1904 through 1973, always seemed to have a populist flavor to it—the intent to deliver accessible, high-quality health care to a large portion of the population at an affordable cost. The two main features have been prepayment and group practice. Throughout the early portions of this chapter, *managed health care* will be used almost interchangeably with *HMO*, because until 1980 the two terms essentially did refer to the same structures and mechanisms. It was only during the 1980s that managed health care truly came to capture broader and more varied health care delivery and reimbursement mechanisms (which we hope that later sections of this chapter will reflect).

Managed Health Care as a National Policy

President Nixon's 1971 Health Message to the Congress was, for all practical purposes, what brought the concept of managed mental health care into modern health policy. The president's expressed goal in his National Health Strategy was to "build a true 'health system'—and not a 'sickness' system alone. We should work to maintain health and not merely to restore it" (Nixon, 1971). This idea was adopted, along with the HMO concept, by the Nixon administration and subsequently expressed in the Health Maintenance Organization Act (HMO Act) of 1973 (PL 93-222).

Federal Legislation on Health Maintenance Organizations

The HMO Act of 1973 provided federal funding for the development of new health maintenance organizations. It also created a certification process, known as *federal qualification,* for HMOs meeting certain financial and organizational standards. The intent of the bill was to provide loans and subsidies in the amount of $325 million over the first 5 years of the initial 10-year plan ("HMO law includes," 1974). The new law superseded some aspects of state law and required that many employees in the United States had to be offered the option of joining an HMO, if they so desired. Any employer with more than 25 employees, subject to the Fair Labor Standards Act, and providing health insurance benefits was required to offer an HMO option as an alternative to its existing health plan, if a federally qualified HMO was available in its area (and the HMO asked to be included).

To qualify for federal subsidies, HMOs were required by law to provide a comprehensive set of eight basic services, including outpatient mental health care and crisis intervention services. Treatment and referral services for alcoholism or drug abuse were also included as basic benefits. Other basic benefits included consultation and referral services, emergency health services, diagnostic laboratory services, diagnostic and therapeutic radiologic services, home health services, and preventive health services (e.g., voluntary family planning, infertility services, preventive dental care for children; "HMO law includes," 1974). Charges for supplemental health services (i.e., long-term nursing care, visual care, prescription drugs) could be billed as a separate expense (Flinn et al., 1987).

In addition to subsidizing the creation and expansion of HMOs, the 1973 HMO Act also allowed the inclusion of profit-making corporations (which were not associated with the HMO movement up to that point) as part of this health program. The law also opened the door to the *medical care foundation,* the forerunner of the independent practice association or IPA (Bennett, 1988).

The restrictive nature of the requirements for federal qualification was modified by amendments in 1976 and 1978. These amendments resulted in further expansion of HMOs (Flinn et al., 1987). The 1976 amendments liberalized HMO requirements and created widespread industry acceptance of federal qualification (National Industry Council for HMO Development, n.d.).

In enacting the Health Maintenance Organization Amendments of 1976 (PL 94-460), the congressional committees with jurisdiction over the program noted that

> Since the Act's inception progress in implementation has been slow . . . [the bill] is intended to correct the identified deficiencies in the original law, improve the administration of the program, and make HMOs meeting the

law's requirements more competitive with traditional insurance programs and health delivery systems. . . . It is clear that some of the requirements of the original Act are excessively strict and have the effect of placing developing HMOs at a competitive disadvantage with other parts of the health care system. This has been demonstrated by a survey by the General Accounting Office (GAO) as a part of its mandated responsibilities under the original Act. (U.S. Senate Report No. 94-884, 1976, pp. 4–6)

Particularly noteworthy for psychology was the General Accounting Office (GAO) finding that the more than 500 organizations surveyed had highlighted the high cost of providing the required basic and supplemental mental health services as a major problem. The 1976 amendments provided greater administrative flexibility for the HMO program, making it more practical for interested groups to become federally qualified. For example, HMOs were allowed to contract for professional services with individual health professionals or groups of health professionals that did not qualify as medical groups or IPAs, provided that the amount contracted for did not exceed a specified value. Similarly, HMOs were authorized to use the clinical expertise of "other health care personnel" (which included nurse practitioners and clinical psychologists for the first time since the program's inception). Modifications were also made to the provisions governing reimbursement under Medicare and Medicaid; these essentially provided that only federally qualified HMOs were eligible for financial support.

The Health Maintenance Organization Act Amendments of 1978 (PL 95-559) were enacted during a period of slow but steady expansion by HMOs, even though there was some evidence of increasing acceptance by the business and labor communities. The resulting congressional view was that further legislative refinement was necessary for the program to become even more competitive in the marketplace (U.S. Senate Report No. 95-837, p. 3). In proposing to reauthorize the program for an additional five years, the Senate committee with jurisdiction noted that

> While HMOs are not the final answer to the health care cost problem, they do give providers strong incentives to reduce unnecessary expenditures; and they create much-needed competition for the health care dollar. HMOs have now proven their cost-saving abilities. We now know that they can achieve overall cost savings of from 10%–40%. Available statistics also show reductions in inpatient hospitalization utilization in an HMO system. Another advantage of HMOs is their ability to deliver health care of high quality and in innovative forms. (U.S. Senate Report No. 95-837, 1978, p. 8)

The conferees ultimately agreed to provide authority for $68 million in fiscal year 1981, significantly more than the $31 million authorized for fiscal year 1979, and to establish a new National Health Maintenance Organization Intern Program to train individuals to become administrators and medical directors or to assume other managerial positions within HMOs. In addition, Congress also found it necessary to require reporting and disclosure of financial information concerning HMOs so as to trigger the Department of Health, Education, and Welfare's (DHEW) monitoring of self-dealing situations. Congress learned of serious abuses in 1975 and wanted to ensure that what it considered to be isolated examples of health care profiteering would not jeopardize the viability of the HMO concept (U.S. Senate Report No. 95-837, p. 12). A delicate balance was sought to prevent abuses of the program without stifling the development of a promising health care reform. The key policy concept was a reliance on disclosure and reporting requirements, rather than a ban on particular activities per se.

This primarily economics-oriented concern about crucial interested parties would turn out to be the forerunner of organized psychology's eventual concern with clinical conflicts of interest, in which HMOs were alleged to provide economic incentives to ensure that even essential care would not be provided, unless absolutely necessary. This latter concern was addressed by the Heinz-Stark proposal, which ultimately was included as a provision of the Omnibus Budget Reconciliation Act of 1986 (OBRA–86; PL 99-509). The provision stipulated that beginning April 1, 1990, an HMO or competitive medical plan (CMP) would be subject to civil penalties if it made a payment to a physician as an inducement to reduce or limit services to beneficiaries enrolled under a contract with Medicare or Medicaid. The proposed civil penalty could be as high as $2,000 for each enrollee for whom such a payment is made. The implementation of this provision was subsequently delayed until April 1, 1991, by the Omnibus Budget Reconciliation Act of 1989 (OBRA–89; PL 101-239), after the House proposed a repeal of the Medicare (but not Medicaid) civil penalty.

The underlying issue of potential conflict, however, did not go away. OBRA–89 also included a provision directing the GAO to conduct a study of ownership of hospitals and other Medicare providers of referring physicians (e.g., laboratories). The conference report explicitly stated that

> The conferees wish to make clear that if the report by GAO finds that referring physician ownership of hospitals and other providers of Medicare items or services or ownership interest in such entities by referring physicians leads to inappropriate use of services or inappropriately alters admission or utilization patterns in favor of entities or services in which physicians have an ownership interest, it would be the intent of the relevant committees to consider legislation banning referrals at the earliest possible date. Investors in entities should take this possibility into account prior to investing in such arrangements. (U.S. House of Representatives Report No. 101-386, 1989, p. 855)

Professional psychology was rightfully pleased with its legislative accomplishment in obtaining autonomous recognition under Part B of Medicare during the 101st Congress. However, relatively few professional psychologists appreciate that psychology obtained its first substantive recognition as an autonomous provider under Medicare when risk-sharing HMOs were authorized to provide the services of clinical psychologists as a provision of the Deficit Reduction Act of 1984 (PL 98-369). Subsequently, the Health Maintenance Organization Amendments of 1986 (PL 99-660) explicitly included psychologists in the list of authorized HMO health professionals. Prior to this modification of the underlying authorization statute, psychologists' services were recognized only under the broad heading of *other health care providers*.

As shown in our earlier discussion of the various HMO amendments, Congress and the administration remain convinced that actively encouraging prepaid and managed health care efforts are in the nation's best interest. The Health Maintenance Organization Amendments of 1988 (PL 100-517) continued the trend of providing appropriate administrative flexibility. With the 1988 amendments, it was decided that it was no longer necessary to require firms with 25 employees or more to specifically provide an HMO health benefit. However, the historical financial nondiscrimination provisions were not repealed. The 1988 amendments also included language that would override state laws and regulations that were deemed to prohibit HMOs from meeting the federal HMO requirements.

The Bush administration's continued support was made quite clear during Health and Human Services Secretary Louis Sullivan's 1991 Senate Appropriations Committee hearings. Sullivan stated that

> Our legislative agenda includes several initiatives which will encourage the provision of health services in managed care settings. We believe managed care is the best means of assuring quality service and appropriate care for Medicare and Medicaid beneficiaries. (Sullivan, 1990; cf. Adler, 1990)

Medicare and the HMO Movement

A new market for HMO plans was created within Medicare by the Tax Equity and Fiscal Responsibility Act of 1982 (TEFRA; PL 97-248). TEFRA made major changes in the way the Medicare program reimburses HMOs. Under the new rules, Medicare beneficiaries could be routinely enrolled in federally qualified HMOs and CMPs (Merlis, 1988).

TEFRA provided that the financial arrangements between Medicare and the HMO under a risk-sharing contract would be comparable to those prevailing in the private sector. The HMO would receive a fixed monthly capitation payment for each enrolled beneficiary and would be fully at risk for the provision of all Medicare-covered services, including physician services, hospital inpatient services, outpatient services, skilled nursing facilities, and home health care.

The TEFRA rules were to take effect when the secretary of Health and Human Services (HHS) certified to Congress that a satisfactory method for establishing premium rates had been developed. From 1982 through 1984, the secretary entered into demonstration contracts with 26 HMO organizations, using a general statutory authority to waive legal requirements in order to test program improvements. By the end of 1984, 117,588 beneficiaries were enrolled in these experiments. In January 1985, the HHS secretary certified that the rate-setting method was ready, and the first TEFRA contracts were made soon after. As of September 1987, 1.1 million of the 22.5 million Medicaid recipients were in HMOs, and in 1990, 1.8 million of the 33.2 million Medicare recipients were in HMOs (Adler, 1990).

The use of HMOs in the Medicare program has not been without problems and criticisms. The potential negative impact on quality of psychological care was noted relatively early in the process of using HMOs with Medicare (Welch, 1986a). The potential for physicians to abuse the economic incentives available to them was also cited (Welch, 1986b). Examples of mismanagement and other administrative problems also attracted early attention (Buie, 1987). Subsequent amendments have aimed at strengthening the monitoring of quality of care and at eliminating alleged abuses in the areas of marketing, enrollment, disenrollment, and financial management (Merlis, 1988).

In its 1991 budget proposal, the Bush administration wanted more Medicare and Medicaid recipients to use managed-care programs (Adler, 1990). The administration proposed legislation to Congress that would increase payments to states for Medicaid recipients in managed-care programs and make it easier for states to require recipients to use HMOs. At the same time, the change would lower premiums of Medicare recipients who enroll in HMOs and increase payments to the HMOs that treat them. Congress and some psychologists opposed the proposal because of continued skepticism about the quality of care currently provided by managed-care programs to Medicaid recipients.

CHAMPUS and Managed Health Care

The Civilian Health and Medical Program of the Uniformed Services (CHAMPUS) within the Department of Defense (DoD) is responsible for providing health care to approximately 2.2 million active-duty personnel and an additional 7 million dependents of active-duty personnel, retirees, and the dependents of retirees and deceased military personnel. The general operational policy has been that, where possible, DoD will provide necessary care through its own facilities and use CHAMPUS (a traditional fee-for-service plan) to purchase care from the private sector only when it is not available through DoD facilities (Uyeda, DeLeon, Perloff, & Kraut, 1987). The department's fiscal year 1991 budget request for health care was $13 billion, of which $2.9 billion was targeted for CHAMPUS.

Between 1981 and 1984 CHAMPUS costs increased 7.3% faster than private sector health costs. CHAMPUS costs rose from $1.2 billion in fiscal year 1984 to approximately $1.8 billion in fiscal year 1986, with no increase in the eligible beneficiary population—a 50% cost increase in 2 years. In fiscal year 1987, for example, DoD reported that CHAMPUS costs had increased by 43% over the fiscal year 1985 level, whereas DoD's internal medical costs (excluding CHAMPUS) had increased only 21.6%. By comparison, during the same time period the nation's overall health care expenditures had increased 18%. During the late 1980s, the DoD began experiencing annual unbudgeted cost overruns of $300 million to $400 million, resulting in a doubling of CHAMPUS costs over a 5-year period.

Dr. William "Bud" Mayer served as assistant secretary for health affairs of the DoD during the Reagan administration. It was his judgment that, in response to the escalating CHAMPUS expenditures, DoD should experiment with a managed-care approach. In December 1985, the DoD proposed a major restructuring of CHAMPUS. The National Defense Authorization Act for fiscal year 1987 (PL 99-661) directed DoD to test out its proposed major managed-care initiative.

In announcing the CHAMPUS Reform Initiative (CRI) in June 1986, DoD noted that

> In recent years, the rate of growth of CHAMPUS costs significantly exceeded that of health care generally in the United States. The average annual rate of growth of CHAMPUS thus far in the 1980s is 45 percent higher than it was in the 1970s . . . . In addition, from 1983 to 1986, the average annual growth rate for CHAMPUS [was] more than one-fifth higher than that for total U.S. health care expenditures. The difference in growth rates is even more dramatic in hospital care expenditures during this period, with the CHAMPUS rate more than 50 percent higher than that of the total U.S. (Mayer, 1986)

The policy notions underlying the CRI program were as follows: (a) The department would be using its nationwide buying power to improve and expand services. (b) The contractor was to be financially at risk, assuming financial responsibility for virtually all health care services provided under CHAMPUS. (c) The contractor would be expected to develop a network of providers who were willing to provide quality care at reduced rates. (d) Priority would be given to providing preventive care and careful clinical management to ensure that individual providers would not be financially encouraged to use more expensive inpatient care or diagnostic testing and clinical interventions, unless absolutely necessary.

The DoD's original plan was to award three such contracts, covering the entire United States. CRI was to address three prime objectives: (a) reducing costs; (b) improving access to quality care, with an emphasis on providing preventive and primary care; and (c) significantly improving the coordination between use of military facilities and CHAMPUS. Under no circumstances were the costs to exceed what the projected CHAMPUS expenditures would have been. Thus, to the extent that the contractor could remain below the projected target cost, his profit could be substantial.

As designed by the DoD, there were to be three basic options available to CHAMPUS beneficiaries, including the right to remain with their current fee-for-service CHAMPUS coverage if the contractor could not convince them of a more attractive alternative.

1. *CHAMPUS Prime.* This was crucial to the success of CRI. Under this option, beneficiaries would annually be given the right to enroll to receive all of their civilian-provided health care from the contractor-established provider network at a substantially lower charge and without any paperwork. Individual beneficiary health care finders were assigned to facilitate appropriate use of the system, and a wide range of preventive care was readily available. Essentially, this represented a contractor-designed HMO.

2. *CHAMPUS Extra.* This option did not require beneficiary preenrollment and offered specialized care, to be provided by the Standard CHAMPUS. The newly established preventive care option was not available. Essentially, this represented a contractor-established PPO (preferred provider organization) model.

3. *Standard CHAMPUS.* The current benefit that was available to all CHAMPUS beneficiaries, with the traditional beneficiary paperwork, copayment and first-dollar charges, and the requirement of certificates of nonavailability for inpatient care, if the beneficiary resided within a specified distance from a military treatment facility.

The underlying concept of the proposal was the establishment of a 3-year phase-in of CRI, starting with a 1-year demonstration (to be followed, if successful, by nationwide implementation). According to DoD, among the most significant improvements that would be made by the proposed CHAMPUS reforms would be increased access to primary care. From the beginning, the department planned to require the contractor to establish primary care centers in areas throughout the United States with overcrowded military hospitals. The primary care to be provided would include family practice, pediatrics, gynecology, and internal medicine, in the context of a normal office-based medical practice. The contractor was also expected to work closely with the various base commanders within the designated catchment area to facilitate the use of military facilities by selected civilian health care providers.

Health care services were first offered through CHAMPUS Prime on August 1, 1988, in nine catchment areas: Beale Air Force Base (AFB), George AFB, March AFB, Mather AFB, Travis AFB, Long Beach Naval Base, San Diego Naval Base, Camp Pendleton Marine Base, and Tripler Army Medical Center. Beginning on March 1, 1989, the areas offering CHAMPUS Prime were expanded to include Oakland Naval Hospital, Letterman Army Medical Center, and Fort Ord. Essentially, CRI covered the states of California and Hawaii.

From the beginning it was quite clear that the CHAMPUS Reform Initiative would have a significant impact on the delivery of mental health care in the areas selected. According to DoD, in 1987 (prior to CRI) mental health costs per CHAMPUS eligible in California and Hawaii were 52% higher than the CHAMPUS national average. Inpatient days and outpatient visits there exceeded the CHAMPUS national average by 27% and 65% respectively. In addition, tremendous cost variations existed within California, with the San Diego area having the highest.

The department's June 1989 report to Congress specifically noted that

> Mental health services comprise an extremely large proportion of total services consumed by CHAMPUS beneficiaries. For example, among patients in the Extra option for the period ending December 31, 1988, mental health bed-days accounted for 24 percent (Northern California) to 98 percent (Hawaii) of all bed-days. Thus, we would expect efforts to curtail inappropriate use of inpatient mental health services to be particularly rewarding. Commensurate with the importance of mental health under CHAMPUS,

> FHC (Foundation Health Corporation, the CRI contractor) is assembling a
> sizable mental health UM (Utilization Management) team. However, un-
> derstaffing remains a problem in some areas. . . . Complaints from mental
> health providers, especially in southern California, allege that mental health
> UM is proceeding inefficiently and resulting in denials of appropriate care.
> Although we receive copies of these complaints and plan in the future to
> interview these and other providers, a thorough investigation of these com-
> plaints is not within the scope of our evaluation. (U.S. Department of De-
> fense, June 1989, p. 16)

The department's December 1989 report to Congress indicated that 12
reports already had been submitted to Congress on the project. California and
Hawaii accounted for approximately 865,000 CHAMPUS beneficiaries, representing 14% of the total CHAMPUS beneficiary population. The contractor
had reported that its CHAMPUS Prime enrollment had reached over 55,000
individuals by October 1989, which was substantially more than expected for
the first 15 months of activity. Between 1988 and 1989, the total costs involved
increased by 4.5%; but in comparison, nationwide (excluding California and
Hawaii) CHAMPUS costs had increased 17%. The report further noted that
"The biggest decrease we found was for professional and outpatient mental
health services. Excluding adjustments, the costs for these services decreased
by an astounding 34 percent" (U.S. Department of Defense, December 1989,
p. 4). Perhaps most important for Congress, the evaluation noted that "Of the
beneficiaries who had formed an opinion about the medical care they received,
97 percent were satisfied. . . . [M]ore than 90 percent of the sample stated they
would recommend the program to a friend" (p. 9).

Although there is no question that CRI had major administrative problems
in its early stages (Buie, 1988; Fisher, 1986), there seems to be somewhat
better acceptance of it now, as stated by the department's newly confirmed
assistant secretary for health, the three service surgeons general, and representatives from military families during their testimony before the Senate
Appropriation Committee hearings in March 1990.

The departmental witnesses at the March 1990 hearings noted that

> The CRI has been delivering services now in California and Hawaii for a
> year and a half. Its impact is definite. Beneficiaries are happy with the
> improved medical benefits from participating providers, not having to file
> their own claims, preventive care, and the system of health care finders.
> Over 11,000 doctors and 130 hospitals have joined networks. 69,000 bene-
> ficiaries are enrolled in CHAMPUS Prime. . . . Military hospital com-
> manders have voiced strong support for the program. Resource sharing
> agreements with the contractor have allowed them to respond to beneficiary
> needs by increasing their in-house capabilities, recapturing CHAMPUS
> workload. CRI provides our military hospital commanders with an easy-to-
> use, cost-effective tool that truly helps them manage the beneficiary pop-
> ulation within their catchment areas at a predictable, fixed price. . . . [T]he
> RAND Corporation found that CRI costs increased 4.6 percent in California
> and Hawaii. . . . With an estimated $30 million savings in two states during
> its first year, that tells me CRI has some features that can dramatically

help our military hospitals and CHAMPUS, with which they interface under CRI, become a more efficient and cost effective integrated health care system. (U.S. Department of Defense, 1990)

Furthermore, the department requested the authority to expand CRI later on in fiscal year 1991 if the results continued to be as promising.

Nonetheless, the congressional committees are carefully observing the implementation of the CRI mental health care projects on the West Coast because of problems involving delays in reimbursement, confusing and contradictory guidelines, increased paperwork, and complaints about unreasonable limitations on inpatient hospitalization and other forms of care (Buie, 1989a). Congressional plans appear to be leaning toward delaying the implementation of CRI initiatives for managed care in Arizona and New Mexico.

Growth of HMOs and Managed-Care Systems

President Nixon hoped to make the HMO option available to 90% of the population through the establishment of 1,700 HMOs over a 10-year period (DeLeon, Uyeda, & Welch, 1985). The reality is that far fewer HMOs came into being. In 1983, 10 years after the passage of the initial federal HMO Act, there were 280 HMOs, covering 12 million Americans, or about 5.1% of the U.S. population (DeLeon, VandenBos, & Kraut, 1984).

Prior to the HMO Act of 1973, the Department of Health, Education, and Welfare (DHEW; now the Department of Health and Human Services, HHS) had been encouraging the development of prepaid health plans. However, the passage of the 1973 legislation allowed the federal government to foster and stimulate HMO growth through a federal grant and loan program. Between 1973 and 1981, the federal government provided a total of $364 million ($145 million in grants and $219 million in loans) for the support and development of 115 operational HMOs—or about 40% of those in operation in 1983 (National Industry Council for HMO Development, n.d.). Under President Carter, HHS evaluated the original HMO plan and initiated a new 10-year plan (1978–1988) targeting the establishment of 450 HMOs, with an enrollment population goal of 20 million by 1988 (DeLeon et al., 1984). By 1988, there were 659 HMOs nationwide, serving about 33.7 million individuals.

The HMO movement has grown and matured since 1973. Managed-care systems are now an established part of the U.S. health care system. In 1970, there were 33 HMOs covering 3 million persons (1.5% of the U.S. population), and, in 1980, there were 236 HMOs serving 9.1 million members—about 4% of the U.S. population (National Industry Council for HMO Development, n.d.). HMO growth continued in the early 1980s, but slowed in the late 1980s. The number of HMOs reached an all-time high of 707 plans in 1987. However, the number of plans decreased in 1988, 1989, and 1990. By the end of 1989, there were 623 operating HMOs, down 5.5% from 1988. The number of operating HMOs was expected to decrease to 612 by the end of 1990, with further decreases projected through 1994, when there will be an estimated 568 plans in operation. The decrease in the number of operating HMOs is explained by industry sources as a reflection of continued consolidation in the industry as HMOs are shut down, become insolvent, or are acquired by other HMOs. However, total enrollments were up 3.9% to 35.03 million (14% of the U.S. population) in 1989, compared with 1988 when 659 HMOs served some 33.7 million members. Enrollments were expected to reach an estimated 36.9 million in 1990 and 53.2 million by the end of 1994 (Marion Laboratories, 1989; Marion Merrel Dow, 1990). Thus, the percentage of the U.S. population actually covered by HMO systems tripled during the 1970s and more than tripled again during the 1980s. However, there are not 50 million or 100 million Americans "trapped" in managed-care systems, as some critics have claimed.

HMOs and managed health care systems ended the 1980s with some uncertainty about their economic and organizational future (Traska, 1990). Between 1985 and 1989, there had been many sizeable annual losses by HMOs, a few consolidations, and a couple of bankruptcies. However, although the HMO industry was viewed as being on somewhat shaky financial ground, annual growth in enrollment was continuing to increase at a rate between 5% and 6%.

The classic model of an HMO was a prepaid group practice (or prepaid staff practice) system. By the late 1970s, there were criticisms of such models by both consumers and providers, which led to the development of loosely contracted individual practice association (IPA) models of managed health care. In the late 1970s and early 1980s, the majority of the new HMOs, which were often strongly physician dominated, followed the IPA model.

Another variation of managed-care and cost-containment mechanisms is the preferred provider organization (PPO). PPO arrangements involve contracts between insurers and providers, whereby the insurer receives discounts on standard provider service rates, the provider is assured referrals (and often a certain volume of business), and utilization review is an active and extensive programmatic feature. There are relatively few stand-alone PPOs, as PPOs are more generally an option available in addition to a standard indemnity plan. Although it is estimated that more than 30 million Americans may be eligible for PPO options, it is unknown how many actually use such features of their health insurance plans (Traska, 1990).

A major national survey of HMOs and managed care was conducted in 1986 (Shadle & Christianson, 1988). One part of the study examined the growth and changes within individual HMOs and within the managed-care industry.

Three major trends were noted by Shadle and Christianson (1988) about the managed health care industry. First, the mix of organizational structures of HMOs has changed. Among HMOs 3 years old or younger, 75% are IPA models. In 1989, IPAs made up about 62% of all HMOs, compared with about 37% in 1981. Second, the HMO industry has undergone a change in the mix of for-profit versus not-for-profit firms. Sixty-two percent of all HMOs in 1987 were for profit, with three fourths of the plans under 3 years of age being for profit. Virtually all new HMOs established in 1988 and 1989 were for profit (Marion Merrel Dow, 1990). Although data on the profit status of HMOs is not consistently available over time, it is evident that the role of the for-profit HMOs has steadily grown. Although not-for-profit HMOs still enroll 60% of all HMO members, enrollment in for-profit HMOs grew by 19% in 1986, compared with a 3% growth rate for not-for-profit plans. Third, there has been a continuing shift in the HMO industry away from small, independent HMOs toward multistate networks of HMOs linked by common ownership and management. In 1986, about 50% of all HMOs were linked to national firms, and these multistate health care firms enrolled 60% of all HMO members. By 1989, 47 multistate HMO chains owned and operated 411 (66%) of HMO plans, enrolling 73.8% of all HMO members in the United States (Marion Merrel Dow, 1990).

Mental Health Care in HMOs

Mental health (or psychological) care is a relatively new addition to HMOs. Despite their commitment to comprehensive care, the prototype HMOs of the 1940s and 1950s did not include benefits or treatment for mental illness. One exception was the St. Louis Labor Institute HMO. The Health Insurance Plan of Greater New York provided only mental health diagnosis and consultation, and Kaiser Permanente provided mental health services on a reduced-fee fee-for-service basis (Bennett, 1988).

In the 1960s, in response to the influence of large contractor groups (e.g., FEHBP, unions and employee groups), HMOs started including mental health care on an optional (rider) basis. New HMO plans that emerged in the late 1960s, such as the Harvard Community Health Plan, included substantial mental health care as a basic benefit (Bennett, 1988).

With the passage of the 1973 HMO Act, prepaid health plans that wished to be federally qualified had to meet the requirements for emergency and outpatient crisis intervention services by providing up to 20 visits per year. Alcohol and substance abuse services were also required ("HMO law includes," 1974). The initial legislation was somewhat imprecise concerning the nature and extent of mandated mental health coverage, and administrative interpretation of this legislation has allowed considerable latitude in services provided (Cheifetz & Salloway, 1984a). This has emerged as a larger and larger problem over time (cf. Buie, 1989c), particularly among IPAs.

The possibilities of overutilization, inappropriate utilization, and runaway costs were early concerns about the inclusion of a mental health component in comprehensive managed health care plans. However, in an evaluation of Kaiser Permanente's experience with psychotherapy and medical utilization, Cummings and VandenBos (1981) showed that the inclusion of mental health benefits within a comprehensive health care plan did not bankrupt the health care financing system. Early in its experience of providing capitated health care, Kaiser Permanente discovered the value of providing mental health services to prevent overutilization of medical facilities by healthy persons who were somatizing. This is now referred to as the *medical offset effect* (Jones & Vischi, 1979; Luft, 1987; Mechanic, 1975; Mumford, Schlesinger, Glass, Patrick, & Cuerdon, 1984; VandenBos & DeLeon, 1988).

The Kaiser Permanente experience showed that the cost of providing quality mental health coverage is not costly or uncontrollable: The average cost

increased 3.5% per year between 1959 and 1979, whereas nationwide general
medical costs increased between 12% and 20% per year (Kiesler, Cummings,
& VandenBos, 1979, p. 206). In addition, the Kaiser Permanente plan demonstrated that mental health utilization rates are predictable and that mental
health is insurable: Utilization rates at Kaiser Permanente rose to a predictable level and remained stable thereafter.

It is critical to a cost-effective managed health care system that there be
multiple entry points for gaining access to psychological care. A single entry
point controlled by one profession with one orientation makes for a costly,
biased, inefficient, and nonresponsive system of care, in part because primary
care providers are not the most able to determine whether psychological care
is needed. When the patient believes he or she should seek psychological treatment, it is appropriate, from both a quality-of-care perspective and a cost-
efficiency basis, to allow him or her to directly seek and obtain needed mental
health services (Cummings & VandenBos, 1981).

The Shadle and Christianson (1988) HMO survey was conducted in the
fall of 1986. It provided a useful overview of the nature of mental health
services currently provided in managed-care systems. The survey form was
sent to 473 HMOs in operation in the United States as of December 31, 1985.
After follow-up mailing and telephone contact, 286 responses were obtained,
for a 60.5% response rate. Newer, smaller, for-profit, non-federally qualified,
or IPA model HMOs were statistically less likely to respond.

Almost 70% of responding HMOs reported that they delivered all or most
of their mental health services internally, with about 47% reporting that they
delivered all of their mental health services internally. Conversely, 17.6% of
HMOs reported using external providers for all or almost all of their mental
health care. Both staff model HMOs (69.2%) and group model HMOs (48.3%)
were more likely to offer all mental health services internally. Likewise, large
HMOs were more likely than smaller HMOs to directly provide mental health
care.

Slightly more than one half of the responding HMOs reported having a
specific mental health director or coordinator—about 42% of whom were psychiatrists, and about 28% were psychologists. Older HMOs and larger HMOs
were more likely to have a mental health director, and IPAs were by far the
least likely to have such a specialty coordinator.

In terms of staffing, HMOs with internal mental health service provision
employed an average of 3.05 psychiatrists per 10,000 enrollees, 1.61 PhD psychologists, and 1.38 psychiatric nurse–social workers. Regardless of the size
of the HMO, more psychiatrists than psychologists were employed in all settings involving covered populations of fewer than 200,000 individuals, although it is not fully clear whether or not these data are reported on a full-
time-employee basis. Although Wiggins (1976) was initially optimistic about
HMOs as potential employment sites for psychologists, HMOs have not emerged
as a major employment setting for psychologists (Cheifetz & Salloway, 1984b).

In the vast majority of HMOs, the primary care physician is the key
referral agent to mental health specialists or specialty units (contrary to Kaiser
Permanente's experience). About 75% of HMOs indicated that the approval of

the patient's primary care physician was required for any alcohol, drug abuse, and mental health (ADM) service to be obtained, although the relative frequency of this requirement varied among types of HMO structures. In general, older, larger, and not-for-profit HMOs were slightly less likely to control mental health access through physician approval than were newer, smaller, and for-profit HMOs. IPA model HMOs were much more likely (88%) to require physician referral than were staff model HMOs (58%). However, this does not mean that self-referral for psychological services is forbidden. Slightly more than one half of the responding HMOs reported that self-referral for mental health care was permissible and that half of all mental health utilization was self-initiated.

Among HMOs using external providers, more than 75% reported using the services of private practitioners for outpatient therapy services. Sixty percent reported that they also had outpatient subcontracts with community mental health centers, and about 45% reported contracts with hospital-based outpatient clinics. For inpatient residential services, more than 85% of HMOs reported contracts with community or general hospitals, and about 70% with private psychiatric hospitals.

The primary outpatient mental health service provided was individual psychotherapy, with 71% of outpatient service being of this type. Group therapy, couples therapy, and family therapy constituted most of the rest of the service. For HMO enrollees utilizing outpatient mental health care, 63% were treated in fewer than 10 sessions; 26% were seen for between 11 and 20 sessions; and 11% had more than 20 sessions. The average length of treatment, by our estimate, was between 9.56 and 11.62 sessions. In terms of inpatient care, 80% of HMO enrollees receiving such care were hospitalized for fewer than 2 weeks.

Although the Shadle and Christianson (1988) HMO survey suggested fairly good availability of psychological services in HMOs, the quality of such care has been questioned (cf. Buie, 1989c), artificial barriers to access to such care has been noted (e.g., Welch, 1986a), and the exclusion of access to psychologist-providers has been legally challenged (Buie, 1990).

Problems and Current Concerns

In the early years of the HMO movement, much of the interest centered on the delivery of accessible, high-quality health care to a fairly large population at an affordable cost. In the view of some, there has been far less attention to HMOs as vehicles for improving quality and access to health care since 1980. In recent years, attention has been concentrated on using HMOs as means of containing costs, providing investment opportunities, and restructuring the medical care system (Luft, 1987; Shulman, 1988; Welch, 1986a, 1986b). The rapid development and proliferation of HMO delivery systems have generated considerable debate and criticism from health care professionals and the public (Buie, 1989b, 1989c; Dorwart, 1990). For example, in Florida, numerous complaints prompted the GAO to conduct an investigation of the new Medicare

HMOs (Welch, 1986a). The GAO found these HMOs to be underregulated by the federal government and that the regulations that did exist were not being enforced—to the detriment of the HMOs' Medicare patients (GAO, 1988).

The primary areas of concern to psychologists in managed-care settings can be categorized into three central issues: access, quality, and consumer–provider awareness (APA Practice Directorate, "Managed Care and Mental Health: Some Potential Problems and Solutions" [internal memorandum], October 30, 1989). Delivery of mental health care and other services to consumers is restricted because of the physician gatekeeping process. Although the Kaiser Permanente experience suggests that patients should have immediate, direct, and easy access to psychological care (for both cost-efficiency reasons and quality-of-care reasons), many HMOs continue to use insensitive mechanisms to attempt to control cost. The use of such gatekeeper referral controls becomes more questionable when the gatekeeper has a financial incentive to block access to needed care (Welch, 1986b). The Omnibus Budget Reconciliation Act of 1986 restricted the use of some such cost-containment mechanisms that provided financial incentives to providers to limit access to care (and possibly lower quality of care).

Managed-care entities often place unrealistic limits on the amount of mental health services provided to clients, either through dollar-amount caps or limits on the number of visits allowed. HMOs and other managed-care operations are not typically structured to provide continuation of mental health treatment once the cap has been exhausted. In addition, a further barrier to mental health services is the increased use of patient copayments being required by HMOs for inpatient mental health and substance abuse services.

The quality and appropriateness of mental health services provided through managed-care systems are often considered inadequate. This problem is demonstrated by the minimal amount of mental health services provided and by the use of a physician gatekeeper who is typically untrained in the mental health area. There is continuing debate on the definition, value, and effectiveness of the short-term (not to exceed 20 visits), outpatient evaluation and crisis intervention mental health services stipulated in the 1973 HMO Act (Buie, 1989c). Because the law is not precise about the nature or extent of mandated mental health services, administrative interpretation of this legislation encourages considerable latitude in services provided. Problems of definition of the outpatient mental health care services that HMOs must provide tend to set limits on participation of all service providers, including psychologists. Individual HMOs may exercise considerable latitude in the eligibility criteria they develop for outpatient mental health services and in the range of such services provided. Thus, the extent and costs of mental health services provided are actually dictated less by law and regulation than by how HMOs interpret and implement them (Cheifetz & Salloway, 1984a). Some psychologists have argued that most HMOs do not provide psychotherapy, as they claim; rather, what HMOs provide are a few hours of "crisis intervention" that is labelled as "psychotherapy" (Buie, 1989c).

In the area of consumer–provider awareness, consumers are often not provided full information about the operation of the managed-care plan and the financial arrangements offered by the managed-care entities. Welch (1986a) has pointed this out as misleading advertising. These entities tend to emphasize only the favorable comparisons between their services and those of traditional health insurance (i.e., that office visits and routine physicals are free, and that there are no deductibles or coinsurance features). Other (negative) features that directly affect access to care and quality of care, such as long delays in scheduling of nonemergency services or excessively time-consuming procedures for applying for psychological care, are not readily apparent to consumers until they want or need such care. In addition, consumers often lack full information about the cost-control mechanisms operating within the managed-care setting. Plans generally do not inform consumers of their use of physician incentive plans that link a provider's decision to refer a patient to a specialist to how much income that physician will receive. The GAO (1988) study of federally qualified HMOs concluded that the practice of HMOs using salary withholding, bonuses, and other incentive arrangements as a way to keep patient care costs down could be jeopardizing the quality of care delivered by HMO plans. These financial arrangements are common throughout the managed-care industry. Likewise, health care providers are often not adequately informed about the managed-care system before they enter into legally binding relationships with HMOs.

Utilization review programs used by most managed-care programs and insurance companies can be problematic in that they employ unlicensed personnel who often receive little training in the field of service they are empowered to review. Moreover, several court cases have indicated that managed-care entities can be found liable for patient injuries resulting from their own negligence. Recent court cases contain language that may be used by courts to find utilization review programs liable in recommending lengths of stay or discharge dates that may harm the patient. Indeed, a third-party payer could be held liable for injuries resulting from an arbitrary or unreasonable decision to deny requests for medical care (APA Practice Directorate, "Managed Care and Mental Health: Some Potential Problems and Solutions" [internal memorandum], October 30, 1989).

The concern with cost containment and the debate on whether HMOs actually reduce health care costs have prompted various studies comparing service and cost variables between HMOs and traditional fee-for-service health care arrangements.

Some of the most important findings in the 1980s have been from the Rand Health Insurance Study (Manning, Leibowitz, Goldberg, Rogers, & Newhouse, 1984). This study was primarily interested in determining whether prepaid group practice delivered less care than the fee-for-service system in situations in which both systems served comparable populations and provided comparable benefits. Rand randomly assigned and compared 1,580 persons who received health care in either one of two types of provider settings in Seattle, Washington: 431 persons were randomly assigned to a fee-for-service physician of their choice, and 1,149 persons to the Group Health Cooperative (GHC) of Puget Sound, a prepaid group practice. In addition, 733 prior enrollees of the GHC served as a control group. Rand was careful in this experiment to address the problem of self-selection that characterized previous studies (i.e., perceived lower costs of services in HMOs may be explained by the fact that each type of system served a different enrollee population). In the Rand study, randomization eliminated most of the opportunities for self-selection, and extensive adjustments were also done to eliminate any remaining sampling bias.

Results showed that the total medical care expenditures for those enrolled in GHC were about 25% lower than expenditures for those in the fee-for-service plan with minimal copayments. This figure resembles comparisons in a variety of similar studies of HMOs, thereby supporting the validity of the findings for the Rand experimental group. The rate of hospital admissions in both groups at GHC was about 40% less than in the fee-for-service group, although the ambulatory visit rate for all services was about 25% less than in the two GHC groups. The number of preventive visits was higher in the prepaid groups, but this difference does not explain the reduced hospitalization. In terms of quality of care, using several measures of health status, the study found that people assigned to GHC did as well as those in the fee-for-service plans, even though they consumed significantly less medical care. A possible explanation for the lower rate of hospitalization was that GHC physicians practiced a less costly style of medicine (i.e., less hospital intensive) than did fee-for-service physicians.

In 1987, Rand began another study, the Medical Outcomes Study (MOS), to assess the quality of health care available at three treatment settings: single-specialty solo or small group practices, HMOs, and large multispecialty group practices—including fee-for-service and prepaid plans (Landers, 1990; Tarlov et al., 1989; Wells, Stewart et al., 1989). The longitudinal study, which will continue through 1991, compiled information on the care received by 22,462 adults in three different treatment settings in Boston, Chicago, and Los Angeles. The MOS examines the relationship between patient outcomes and different treatment settings for patients with one or more of four chronic conditions that commonly affect adults: hypertension, coronary heart disease, diabetes, and depression. Of the 523 health care providers who participated in the study, 74 were clinical psychologists. Other providers included internists, family practitioners, cardiologists, endocrinologists, diabetologists, and psychiatrists.

In terms of mental health care, the study estimated clinicians' awareness of depression for 650 patients with current depressive disorder who received care in each of the three treatment settings (Landers, 1990; Wells, Hays et al., 1989). Results showed that depression was more likely to be detected among depressed patients who visited mental health specialists than among those who visited medical clinicians. Depending on the setting, between 78% and 87% of depressed patients who visited mental health specialists were properly diagnosed, compared with 46% to 51% of depressed patients who visited medical clinicians. Among mental health specialists, 94% of those in large multispecialty group practice identified the depression, compared with 87% of those in solo practice and 78% of those in HMOs. By contrast, 51% of medical clinicians in solo practice detected the depression, 46% of those in HMOs, and 44% of those in large multispecialty group practice.

The type of payment had no significant effect on the likelihood of depressive disorder being detected or treated among patients of mental health specialists. However, among patients of medical clinicians, those receiving prepaid care were significantly less likely to have their depression detected or treated during the visit than were depressed patients receiving fee-for-service care.

Philosophical Concerns for Psychology

Professional psychology is a relatively young profession, having obtained independent licensure in all jurisdictions less than 18 years ago. Although clinical psychologists are steadily increasing in numbers, psychology's 57,500 licensed health care providers (in 1990) are a small number when compared with the 506,000 licensed physicians who are involved in delivering health care in our nation (or the 5,090,100 physicians who are practicing worldwide).

Relatively few psychologists understand the nuances of an integrated health delivery system, and the majority of psychologists have little or no practical experience working within the various managed-care models. One reason for this is that most psychological training institutions have developed isolated rather than integrated practice models. Thus, psychology students do not routinely interact with their colleagues in the various medical specialties (e.g., nursing, optometry, podiatry). As a relatively young and behavioral science-oriented profession, clinical psychology services may seem alien or suspect to those more established disciplines that form the dominant component of current managed-care systems.

As the nation's health delivery systems are forced to become increasingly cost conscious (primarily for economic reasons), psychology's traditional training approach (of ignoring cost factors when determining the best clinical regimen for the patient) becomes increasingly untenable. As one concrete example, the profession of psychology and psychological training institutions have not addressed the issue of systematically using psychological extenders or psychological assistants. Psychologists assume, especially during training experiences, that doctoral-level psychologists should personally perform each phase of the testing protocol, a practice that ignores the experiences of dentistry and medicine.

Clearly, there are similar problems within certain elements of organized medicine. Historically, organized medicine initially attempted to eliminate virtually all prepayment-based managed-care initiatives. Today, the major difference between medicine and psychology is that managed health care systems are controlled and maintained by medicine. The assumption is that HMOs and PPOs must have significant numbers of physicians and nurses to ensure quality health care under these new cost-containment initiatives. Psychologists, on the other hand, at times seem uncomfortable in assuming that their clinical services are a necessary component of health care. Furthermore, although psychology professes to be a data-driven, objective-oriented profession, many senior psychologists are uncomfortable in assuming accountability for their services being safe, effective, and appropriate, as required by federal statute for all drugs and medical devices.

As the profession of psychology matures, and as psychologists become increasingly involved in managed-care programs (general health programs, military health services, etc.), psychology, like medicine and dentistry, will be split. Certain elements of organized psychology will become vocal proponents of managed care; other elements will remain skeptical (at best). We hope that psychologists will demand, and rely on, objective evidence regarding the true clinical consequences of any particular financing system. This is what the controversy surrounding managed care is all about.

References

Adler, T. (1990, April). HMO fever: Bush budget spotlights managed health care. *APA Monitor, 21*, pp. 17–18.

Bennett, M. J. (1988). The greening of the HMO: Implications for prepaid psychiatry. *American Journal of Psychiatry, 145*, 1544–1549.

Buie, J. (1987, September). Evidence of HMO flaws mounting. *APA Monitor, 18*, p. 45.

Buie, J. (1988, January). CHAMPUS project draws mixed reviews. *APA Monitor, 19*, p. 18.

Buie, J. (1989a, June). CHAMPUS programs experience shake-ups. *APA Monitor, 20*, p. 18.

Buie, J. (1989b, June). Given lemons, they make lemonade. *APA Monitor, 20*, p. 20.

Buie, J. (1989c, November). Managed care debate covers pros and cons. *APA Monitor, 20*, p. 21.

Buie, J. (1990, March). HMO's quality of care challenged by lawsuits. *APA Monitor, 21*, p. 13.

Cheifetz, D. I., & Salloway, J. C. (1984a). Mental health services in health maintenance organizations: Implications for psychology. *Professional Psychology: Research and Practice, 15*, 152–164.

Cheifetz, D. I., & Salloway, J. C. (1984b). Patterns of mental health services provided in HMOs. *American Psychologist, 39*, 495–502.

Cummings, N. A., & VandenBos, G. R. (1981). The twenty years Kaiser-Permanente experience with psychotherapy and medical utilization: Implications for national health policy and national health insurance. *Health Policy Quarterly, 1*, 159–175.

DeLeon, P. H., Uyeda, M. K., & Welch, B. L. (1985). Psychology and HMOs: New partnership or new adversary? *American Psychologist, 40*, 1122–1124.

DeLeon, P. H., VandenBos, G. R., & Kraut, A. G. (1984). Federal legislation recognizing psychology. *American Psychologist, 39*, 933–946.

DeLeon, P. H., Willens, J. G., Clinton, J. J., & VandenBos, G. R. (1988). The role of the federal government in peer review. In G. Stricker & A. Rodriguez (Eds.), *Quality assurance in mental health: A comprehensive handbook* (pp. 285–309). New York: Plenum.

Dorwart, R. A. (1990). Managed mental health care: Myths and realities in the 1990s. *Hospital and Community Psychiatry, 41*, 1087–1091.

Fisher, K. (1986, December). Continued role seen in CHAMPUS. *APA Monitor, 17*, p. 29.

Flinn, D. E., McMahon, T. C., & Collins, M. F. (1987). Health maintenance organizations and their implications for psychiatry. *Hospital and Community Psychiatry, 38*, 255–263.

General Accounting Office. (1988). *Medicare physician incentive payments by prepaid health plans could lower quality of care.* (GAO/HRD-89-29). Washington, DC: U.S. Government Printing Office.

HMO law includes mental health services as basic benefit. (1974). *Hospital and Community Psychiatry, 25*, 257–261.

Jones, K. R., & Vischi, T. R. (1979). Impact of alcohol, drug abuse, and mental health treatment on medical care utilization. *Medical Care, 17*(12), 1–82.

Kiesler, C. A., Cummings, N. A., & VandenBos, G. R. (Eds.). (1979). *Psychology and national health insurance: A sourcebook*. Washington, DC: American Psychological Association.

Landers, S. (1990, April). HMO MDs overlook depression. *APA Monitor, 21*, p. 16–17.

Levin, B. L., & Glasser, J. H. (1984). A national survey of prepaid mental health services. *Hospital and Community Psychiatry, 35*, 350–355.

Luft, H. S. (1987). *Health maintenance organizations: Dimensions of performance*. New Brunswick, NJ: Transaction Books.

Manning, G., Leibowitz, A., Goldberg, G. A., Rogers, W. H., & Newhouse, J. P. (1984). A controlled trial of the effect of a prepaid group practice on use of services. *The New England Journal of Medicine, 310*, 1505–1510.

Marion Laboratories. (1989, October). *Marion managed care digest update*. Kansas City, MO: Author.

Marion Merrel Dow. (1990). *Marion managed care digest—HMO edition*. Kansas City, MO: Author.

Mayer, W. (1986, June 16). Letter to members of Congress.

Mechanic, D. (1975). The organization of medical practice and practice orientation among physicians in prepaid and nonprepaid primary care settings. *Medical Care, 13*, 189–204.

Merlis, M. (1988). Medicare: Risk contracts with health maintenance organizations and competitive medical plans. Washington, DC: Congressional Research Service Report for Congress, the Library of Congress.

Mumford, E., Schlesinger, H. J., Glass, G. V., Patrick, C., & Cuerdon, T. (1984). A new look at evidence about reduced cost of medical utilization following mental health treatment. *American Journal of Psychiatry, 141*, 1145–1158.

National Industry Council for HMO Development. (n.d.). *The health maintenance organization industry ten year report, 1973–1983: "A history of achievement, a future with promise."* Washington, DC: Author.

Nixon, R. (1971). Special message to the Congress proposing a National Health Strategy. In *Public papers of the Presidents of the United States* (pp. 170–186). Washington, DC: U.S. Government Printing Office.

Shadle, M., & Christianson, J. B. (1988). Organization of mental health care delivery in HMOs. *Administration in Mental Health, 15*, 201–225.

Shulman, M. E. (1988). Cost containment in clinical psychology: Critique of Biodyne and the HMO. *Professional Psychology: Research and Practice, 19*, 298–307.

Sullivan, L. (1990). Testimony before the Defense Subcommittee of the Senate Appropriations Committee, March 1990. Unpublished.

Tarlov, A. R., Ware, J. E., Jr., Greenfield, S., Nelson, E. C., Perrin, E., & Zubkoff, M. (1989). The medical outcomes study: An application of methods for monitoring the results of medical care. *Journal of the American Medical Association, 262*, 925–930.

Traska, M. (1990). *Managed care 1990: Strong vital signs, uncertain prognosis*. Washington, DC: Faulkner & Gray's Health Care Information Center.

U. S. Department of Defense. (1989, June). *Supplemental report to Congress on the CHAMPUS Reform Initiative Demonstration Project*.

U. S. Department of Defense. (1989, December). *Report to Congress on the CHAMPUS Reform Initiative Demonstration Project*.

U. S. Department of Defense. (1990, March). Testimony before the Labor-Health and Human Services Subcommittee of the Senate Appropriations Committee. Unpublished.

U. S. House of Representatives Report No. 101-386. (1989, November 21). *Omnibus Budget Reconciliation Act of 1989* (conference report to accompany H. R. 3299). 101st Congress, 1st Session.

U. S. Senate Report No. 94-884. (1976, May 14). *Health Maintenance Organization Amendments of 1975*. (Report to accompany H. R. 9019). 94th Congress, 2nd Session.

U. S. Senate Report No. 95-837. (1978, May 15). *Health Maintenance Organization Act Amendments of 1978*. (Report to accompany S. 2534). 95th Congress, 2nd Session.

Uyeda, M. K., DeLeon, P. H., Perloff, R., & Kraut, A. G. (1987). Financing mental health services: A comparison of two federal programs. *American Behavioral Scientist, 30*, 90–110.

VandenBos, G. R., & DeLeon, P. H. (1988). The use of psychotherapy to improve physical health. *Psychotherapy, 25*, 335–343.

Welch, B. (1986a, October). Professional point. *APA Monitor, 17,* p. 35.

Welch, B. (1986b, December). Professional point. *APA Monitor, 17,* p. 30.

Wells, K. B., Hays, R. D., Burnam, M. A., Rogers, W., Greenfield, S., & Ware, J. E., Jr. (1989). Detection of depressive disorder for patients receiving prepaid or fee-for-service care: Results from the medical outcomes study. *Journal of the American Medical Association, 262,* 3298–3302.

Wells, K. B., Stewart, A., Hays, R. D., Burnam, M. A., Rogers, W., Daniels, M., Berry, S., Greenfield, S., & Ware, J. (1989). The functioning and well-being of depressed patients: Results from the medical outcomes study. *Journal of the American Medical Association, 262,* 914–919.

Wiggins, J. G. (1976). The psychologist as a health professional in the health maintenance organization. *Professional Psychology, 7,* 9–13.

3

Basic Issues in Managed Mental Health Services

*Robert J. Resnick, Robert W. Bottinelli,
Marilyn Puder-York, Beatrice Harris,
and Beth Egan O'Keefe*

By all accounts, the traditional form of mental health care delivery, whereby patients are free to choose their providers and third-party payors assume most of the financial risk, is on the decline. In its place, a wide array of so-called alternative health care delivery systems have emerged, called collectively, "managed health care" systems. One of the primary aims of managed-care systems is to control costs, using a variety of cost-containment and cost-shifting mechanisms, including requiring the patient to pay a greater share of the cost of care, placing a cap on benefits received by third-party payors, and limiting the choice of providers to a preselected group. As providers, psychologists[1] need to be aware of the clinical and financial implications of these emerging systems in order to function effectively and influence the design of such systems.

This chapter has three major sections. In the first section, we describe the basic types of managed-care systems, and in the second we delineate the ways in which psychologists may participate in them. In the last section, we discuss the various professional relationship and professional practice issues that affect providers who work in these settings.

An Overview of the Four Most Common Managed-Care Systems

Health Maintenance Organizations

A health maintenance organization (HMO) is an organized system of health care that enlists the services of hospitals, physicians, and other professionals to provide all medically necessary health care, including mental health, for a defined population, typically in return for a capitated payment. HMO health

We gratefully acknowledge the useful comments and other contributions made by Shirley Ann Higuchi, Rodney L. Lowman, and several anonymous reviewers.

[1]Throughout this chapter, the term *psychologist(s)* should, for the most part, be read as being synonymous with *mental health professional(s)*.

care services are arranged and provided to employers or individuals who are the subscribers of the HMO for a fixed, prepaid charge. This prepaid charge made on behalf of the subscribers entitles them to all benefits provided by that system, which may vary from a legally defined minimum, to some more extensive array of services. Psychologists may be employed by HMOs as salaried providers of services, or they may, individually or in a group, contract with HMOs to provide mental health services on a fee-for-service basis.

HMOs originated, not as a means of making profits, but as a means of providing care to underserved populations (see chapter 2 in this book). HMOs have been perceived as containing costs effectively, and their popularity has grown dramatically since 1970. In that year, there were approximately 30 HMOs serving 3 million enrollees. As HMOs were growing, so were health costs increasing. In 1985 it was reported that health care costs in the United States totaled over $425 billion and that, by 1990, health care costs would be consuming 14% of the nation's gross national product.

By their charter, HMOs are established to offer comprehensive care, providing for all the health and mental health needs of their subscribers. They were intended to encourage preventative care in order to keep their clientele more healthy (and also as a cost-cutting measure). Because subscribers pay a capitated fee that is independent of the amount of services received, and because HMOs by law must accept enrollees without regard to prior health status, HMOs have a financial incentive to control services such as specialty care or mental health services. However, the twin goals of cost containment and quality care must be balanced if the HMO is to be effective, and few service providers would ethically base referral or treatment decisions on cost factors alone. There are at least four HMO models: staff, group, network/direct contract, and the individual practice association (IPA). Of the HMO types, the staff model might be expected to maintain the highest level of direct cost control, whereas the IPA model usually maintains the lowest level of cost containment, and the other models fall somewhere between these two extremes.

The staff-model HMO employs providers directly at an HMO-owned facility and compensates the providers with a basic salary that may be supplemented with bonuses based on the HMO's performance and profits. The staff model is considered a "closed panel," that is, services are primarily provided by salaried HMO staff, and outside providers cannot simply sign up to offer their services. Similarly, the group model is considered a closed panel because subscribers may seek care only from a specific, finite number of providers. In the group model, the HMO contracts with either single- or multiple-provider groups as sole purveyors of particular services to the subscribers of that organization. If necessary, the sole providers may contract with other providers for specialty referral. The group model generally has no central facility of its own but rather utilizes the professional provider's office, clinics, or facilities in exchange for a capitated fee for each HMO subscriber assigned to that provider. The per-subscriber fee remains constant, regardless of the number of professional visits made. The professional group decides on its own how those fees are to be disbursed among their providers. In this model, as with capitated systems more generally, a provider may have an incentive to min-

imize outside consultation and referral to specialty providers such as psychologists, because that provider must pay for the additional consultation out
of the fee received from the HMO. However, the cost-cutting incentive must
be paired with the need for quality care. Because subscribers usually can leave
an HMO at least annually, the system cannot consider costs alone in making
treatment decisions and expect to keep subscribers over the long run.

The network/direct contract model is a variation of the group model in
that the HMO contracts directly with individual providers or small professional
groups to provide services to HMO subscribers in the provider's office. Individual providers are reimbursed according to a maximum fee schedule or on
a capitation basis. In this model, many more individual providers are brought
into the HMO network, and there is less reliance on clinics or large, multispecialty practices. The model appears to be more common in rural areas. In
addition, the network/direct contract model is often referred to as an "open
panel" because providers from the surrounding community have ample opportunity to participate.

The IPA model is also considered to be an open-panel HMO. IPAs contract
with a large number of providers recruited either through professional associations or by individual practitioners. Patients are seen in the provider's office,
and the providers are reimbursed on either a fee-for-service or a capitated
basis. In turn, the IPA contracts with a full-service HMO on a capitated basis,
and the IPA provides the services to the HMO members. Often a portion of
the provider's fees are withheld and paid to the provider only if certain utilization target and cost-containment goals are met. As is the case in any
capitation model, IPA providers have a disincentive to refer to specialty service
providers such as psychologists.

Many HMOs, originally organized as nonprofit entities, have converted
to for-profit status, allowing them to obtain potential profits in the competitive
marketplace and to seek additional sources of funds through the issuance of
stock. However, although the federal government has supported HMO con-
versions, state law requirements and regulatory procedures have sometimes
made the conversion process lengthy, complicated, and expensive.

The original federal Health Maintenance Organization Act of 1973, as
amended, provided the legal and financial impetus necessary to develop HMOs
on a national scale. Prior to its enactment, the laws in many states served as
a barrier to HMO development. In some instances, HMOs were classified as
insurance companies and, therefore, were required to maintain substantial
cash reserves as a condition of licensure and were subject to premium taxes.

In addition to state law barriers to HMO development, there have been
significant economic barriers as well. To establish an HMO, the founders needed
to conduct feasibility studies and to fund development costs and initial operating losses. Funds were often unavailable because private investors were
unwilling to invest in what may have been viewed as a new concept and in a
new organization that did not have proven profitability. The HMO Act removed
the legal obstacles to establishing HMOs by preempting state law restrictions
and easing economic burdens through a federal grant and loan program.

Although the federal grant program was discontinued in 1981 and the loan program in 1983, the federal government continues to grant "qualified" status to HMOs meeting comprehensive standards. In return, qualified status provides a potential marketing advantage, because all employers of 25 or more persons must offer their employees an opportunity to enroll in a federally qualified HMO as an alternative to the employer's existing health insurance program if requested or mandated to do so by a federally qualified HMO operating within the relevant service area. Moreover, if more than one HMO exercises this right, then the employer must offer its employees one federally qualified HMO that is organized according to either the IPA or direct contract/ network model, as well as one organized according to either the staff or group model. This statutory requirement is commonly referred to as the "dual-choice" provision, and many states have included similar provisions in their laws.

Closed-panel HMOs generally require that services be obtained only from health professionals employed by the HMO. In contrast, the open-panel HMO is designed to allow broader opportunity for participation by community providers. Some HMOs have failed, at least in part, because federal subsidies or loans are no longer available. HMOs bid for contracts based on a cost estimate of the provided necessary services. The HMO then charges a flat fee (capitation) per subscriber. If the HMO cost estimates are not on target, the HMO may experience fiscal problems, especially if it pays providers on a fee-for-service basis. However, contract rates can be renegotiated annually or semiannually, and large corporations may be able to afford to sustain short-term losses to increase long-term market share and subsequent profitability.

Different structures have been developed to reduce the financial risk of open-panel HMOs. For example, the use of a primary-care physician-gatekeeper serves as a referral and screening mechanism so that the provision of services by the HMO can be controlled in some fashion. In addition, the HMO may capitate its providers by giving them a fixed fee per month, for which the provider agrees to provide all necessary services. In certain instances, they may capitate the employer group by using the cost per enrollee but pay the provider on a fee-for-service basis and withhold 10% or 20% of the fees until the end of the contract period. The provider in this instance may receive the 10% or 20% only if the HMO stayed within the capitated amount. Most HMOs maintain an active utilization and review process to reduce unnecessary utilization and excessive costs and to review patients' satisfaction and quality of care.

Few HMOs appear to offer more than the minimal, mandated mental health benefits required by their national charters or state laws. The gatekeeper model, in which a professional, often a medical generalist, controls access to, length of, and, sometimes, type of, treatment, has been a special problem for psychologist-providers. In some managed-care systems, the gatekeeper model has worked very poorly; at best, in such systems, it has been an encumbrance, requiring the psychologist regularly to justify continuance of treatment to the gatekeeper, who is frequently a nonpsychiatric physician. In such settings, patients may be prevented from getting needed care, and the gatekeeper method of reducing unnecessary cost to the HMO may backfire. In some HMOs, the gatekeeper requirement has proved to forge genuine collegial bonds between nonpsychiatric physicians and psychologist-providers. Referrals to psychologists may actually increase if physicians become more knowledgeable about the benefits to their patients of psychological care.

Closed-panel HMOs are designed so that subscribers can receive services only from professionals employed by the HMO. There are generally two recognized types of closed-panel HMOs: the staff model and group model. The staff model generally employs providers directly at an HMO-owned facility and compensates them with a salary and a bonus based on the HMO's cost performance. In a group model, the HMO contracts with a single or limited number of large multispecialty physician groups to provide medical services to the HMO's members through the group's existing clinics or facilities in exchange for a fixed monthly fee for each HMO member assigned, known as a capitation fee, regardless of the number of patient contacts. The individual physicians are then paid according to the medical group's established practices.

HMOs are obliged by their respective state laws (typically administered by the state's department of insurance) and in their contracting arrangements to provide all necessary medical services, although certain exclusionary provisions may apply. Thus, if the costs for providing care exceed the estimated projected expenses, the HMO could face insolvency problems. HMOs must have catastrophic reinsurance capabilities that will cover unexpectedly heavy losses for member providers. Alternatively, HMOs can have a relationship with an insurance company whereby they pay premiums to guard against catastrophic loss problems. At a certain level of loss, often $35,000 to $50,000 per event, the insurance company will cover the remaining costs. To justify insurance coverage, HMOs must be able to perform statistical computations to arrive at reasonable capitation figures and to maintain sufficient support staff to run the operation, perform utilization review, and bill and review payments. However, psychologists have not, ordinarily, found the ownership of full-service, medically based HMOs to be feasible; HMOs have tended to be medically controlled because the federal HMO law mandates the involvement of physicians but not of psychologists.

"Medical groups" and "individual practice associations" were included in the original HMO model. Physicians were necessary to implement the mandated services, which were to include up to 20 short-term outpatient evaluation and therapy sessions for mental health problems. Clinical psychologists were among the recognized health professionals but were not essential to the original HMO model presented.

Preferred Provider Organizations

A preferred provider organization (PPO) can be described as a health care financing and delivery program that provides financial incentives for consumers to utilize a select panel of preferred providers. The amount paid to the provider is generally a specified percentage below the customary and reasonable rate for the provision of such services. A PPO usually does not assume the underwriting risk of the services but functions more typically as an administrative marketing organization. Hence, a PPO usually serves as a broker between groups of subscribers and providers. However, in the event that a group of professionals forms a PPO, the group may accept the underwriting risk, which is the difference between the subscribers' fees to the PPOs and the cost of the PPO's professional services. A PPO can also be a locally or regionally based system. Regardless of the services provided, each member of the PPO has a contractual arrangement with that provider organization by which the provider agrees to accept a fee that is typically less than the customary charge.

There are two types of PPOs: provider-based and third-party-sponsored, but each has many variants. The provider-based PPO involves a group of providers who offer services for a negotiated and discounted fee. Ordinarily, psychologists who are preferred providers work out of their own offices and are paid on a fee-for-service basis at a negotiated rate. The advantages to the psychologist potentially include a steady flow of referred patients and the certainty of prompt payment. Psychologists are also permitted to sit on boards of directors that set PPO policy. A broker or insurance company puts together a package of mental health services, identifying and contracting with providers who will accept discounts, and markets this package to payors—usually employers. In provider-based PPOs, psychologists can serve as brokers and thereby participate in profits. IPAs can be brokers as well. Usually, PPO subscribers use the preferred provider, but they may see others at a higher fee. A second form of PPO is a third-party-sponsored PPO, wherein a third party negotiates contracts between payors and providers.

Many permutations of PPOs have evolved as the concept has become more accepted in the health insurance market. For example, exclusive provider organizations (EPOs) require that consumers be locked into a group of preferred providers for a period designated in the term of a subscriber certificate, thus reducing the consumers' flexibility to receive coverage for clinical services provided by nonparticipating providers. Likewise, EPOs will not contribute any part of the professional fee to outside providers. A managed-premium PPO (MPPO) is another type of PPO that introduces an element of risk sharing by and between purchasers and providers of service. Although providers are compensated on a fee-for-service basis, a portion of fees is withheld and returned to purchasers if the providers are unable to control utilization. Likewise, the fees paid to providers are oftentimes discounted on the basis of the volume of services delivered by a purchaser under a contractual arrangement with the providers.

Many additional variations of PPO arrangements will emerge as purchasers become more concerned about the introduction of risk sharing into fee-for-service arrangements as an incentive for controlling utilization and expenditures for health care services. Some PPOs, under a "withholding arrangement," take a percentage of the reduced fee. If cost-cutting goals are reached, the withheld funds are distributed to the providers as a bonus or incentive. PPOs also operate somewhat differently from HMOs in that, at least historically, they have not used gatekeepers. Instead, a member selects a provider from a preferred provider list, thereby incurring no copayment. The member can select a provider outside of the select panel; however, the member is generally responsible for the difference between what the PPO pays for the service and the provider's fee. This may serve as a disincentive for the member to go outside the network of the PPO.

Employee Assistance Programs

Although sometimes not considered to be managed-care entities, employee assistance programs (EAPs) are in fact an early and rather widespread example of managed mental health care. EAPs represent a wide variety of program models and services. Most commonly, EAPs provide professional and confidential problem assessment, crisis intervention, brief counseling, and referral to private and community resources for employees and their families to help them resolve or manage problems originating from stress in the workplace or at home. In addition, EAPs may provide personal counseling for stress-related, psychological, and substance abuse problems. EAPs may also offer educational programs to address health promotion and life-style issues that are relevant to the workplace or occupations of a particular group of employees. Finally, EAPs may provide individual or group consulting and training services to management for a broad range of work-related mental health issues.

One of the objectives of EAPs is to reduce the financial and organizational impact of otherwise undetected and untreated employee problems. By early identification, prompt treatment, and making available a support structure to maintain or restore occupational effectiveness, EAPs aim to assist potentially problematic employees and their employers. The EAP may refer out cases requiring longer term mental health care or a different type of intervention.

EAPs are typically capitated programs in which certain types and amounts of mental health services are provided to employees and their family members. EAPs often contract with independent providers, including psychologists, or groups to deliver services, which may be provided either at the employment site or in the provider's office. In more recent models, EAPs may also serve as gatekeepers for other mental health benefits, such as longer term care under the mental health benefit insurance plan.

EAPs can be separated into two major models of service delivery: internal and external. Depending on the model, staff can be composed of a mix of mental health professionals, paraprofessionals, and, in some cases, nonprofessionals. Psychologists can function as either program administrators or providers. In the internal model, services are offered on or nearby the premises of the work environment by staff who are directly employed by the organization or by on-site independent consultants under company contract. The internal EAP is commonly structurally housed within a department associated with human resources. Easy accessibility to the physical location can help increase program visibility and employee participation, although it is important that personal identity and acoustical privacy be maintained in such arrangements. Although employees may be reluctant, initially, to trust the internal EAP because they fear that management will have access to information about them, this resistance is usually overcome once an internal EAP's credibility and reputation for adherence to a strict and well-defined confidentiality policy have been established.

With the external model, services can be provided by one practitioner or a group of independent practitioners, private consulting firms, or nonprofit social service or mental health agencies. Hours of operation are defined by contract between the employer and the external provider. Services are usually available at the offices of the consultant, but may also be provided on company premises. The external program can include most of the same professional services as the internal program; however, the professionals working on site may have an advantage in that they may be more familiar with the internal culture and the sources of work-related stress specific to an organization. The latter difference highlights one of the important tasks for external providers, namely, learning the culture of the organization.

EAPs were originally created in the 1920s primarily to provide intervention and referral for employees with substance abuse problems. However, their spectrum of services has broadened to include a wide range of services for employees and their families as well. The most common EAP is one that provides assessment and brief counseling, followed, theoretically and when clinically necessary, by referral to providers in the community who provide specialized services and longer term treatment. However, patients may often choose to receive only the (generally free) services available through the EAP, either by not seeking outside referral, or by not following through with a referral made. EAPs benefit businesses in several ways. By acting as gatekeepers to mental health services, they have helped businesses control costs. More important, treatment has resulted in increased productivity and job satisfaction and decreased absenteeism. In EAPs that provide management consultation, providers, including psychologists, may consult on the development of health- and mental health-related policies (e.g., AIDS, drug abuse, and dependent care), health and wellness promotion programs, managed-care systems, and mental health benefits. Psychologists may also advise management on strategies for dealing with major involuntary job loss or changes with their employees.

To be perceived as credible by both the sponsoring business organizations and employee-clients, psychologists need to cultivate a variety of skills in addition to traditional clinical assessment and psychotherapy. The EAP's decisions to refer a client for psychotherapy to community providers or to provide short-term counseling directly are based on a clinical assessment of the individual client's presenting problems. EAP staff usually provide only brief and time-fixed counseling; therefore, providers are expected to be able to identify problems and propose appropriate treatment quickly. Typically, a client who is identified for short-term counseling is a person who is experiencing temporary distress in response to unexpected job or personal life-related stressors. Although EAPs expect providers to have excellent diagnostic skills, the use of formal assessment tools (e.g., psychological testing) is often not required.

In addition to providing counseling to company employees and their families, EAP psychologists may also act as an information link and source of referrals to either internal or company-based resources. These resources may address consumer and legal problems; child care and aged parent concerns; or housing, financial, education, and career issues. Psychologists often sponsor seminars and workshops on lifestyle topics (e.g., parenting or caring for elderly relatives), health promotion concerns (stress management), and transition planning (coping with job loss and preretirement). Education efforts for managers may include training individual managers to cope with troubled staff and advising managers on the development of company policy related to mental health concerns of the workforce (e.g., AIDs and drug abuse).

Competitive Medical Plans

Although we will not discuss psychologists' involvement with competitive medical plans (CMPs) in further detail, we include a description here because psychologists need at least to be aware of this type of health care entity. CMPs are HMOs that are qualified and licensed to provide services to Medicare beneficiaries, in accordance with the Tax Equity and Fiscal Responsibility Act (TEFRA) of 1982. Prior to this law's enactment, HMOs generally did not treat many Medicare patients. Most HMOs that provided care to Medicare patients were paid on a traditional Medicare fee-for-service basis geared toward the reasonable cost of providing services. However, many HMO managers and providers were not satisfied with this payment structure because there were no adequate incentives to treat the Medicare population in the same way the HMOs treated the commercial population, that is, on a prepaid basis with appropriate incentives for cost-efficient care. Accordingly, for a number of years the HMO industry lobbied Congress for changes in Medicare reimbursement principles to allow a fixed payment for Medicare beneficiaries enrolled in HMOs. HMOs finally achieved that goal when Congress adopted TEFRA. One important aspect of the TEFRA legislation was that Congress mandated that HMOs would have to use cost savings to benefit Medicare enrollees.

The TEFRA legislation provides that only federally qualified HMOs and CMPs are eligible to provide prepaid services to Medicare beneficiaries on an "at-risk" basis. It was in this context that, for the first time, the term *competitive medical plan* appeared. Although it is clear that the CMP is something other than a federally qualified HMO, the legislation does not provide additional guidance as to what a CMP is. However, at a minimum, a CMP must meet the following criteria: (a) be organized under state law; (b) provide or arrange for a minimum range of health care services; (c) provide these services primarily through physicians who are employees, partners, or contractors of the CMP; (d) assume the financial risk (although CMPs are allowed to buy reinsurance and other financial protection); (e) provide adequate protection for enrollees in the event of insolvency; and (f) be compensated at predetermined rates for the enrolled members.

Professional Participation Options for Psychologists in Managed-Care Entities

Psychologists as Owners

Although the first HMOs were created to satisfy social needs (see chapter 3), as they have grown and become successful, some, such as Kaiser Permanente and some Blue Cross HMOs, have become major corporations with considerable financial resources. Burgeoning expansion of HMOs in the 1980s resulted in a highly competitive marketplace; some HMOs went bankrupt, whereas others merged or were taken over. Because the surviving HMOs are typically large and well capitalized, ownership in any of these corporate entities, other than owning stock in one that is publicly traded, is an unlikely option for most psychologists. Furthermore, ownership in medically based HMOs—those pre-paid health plans offering a full range of medical services, including mental health services—is unlikely because of the substantial start-up costs required. Open-panel HMOs typically require more capital and reinsurance than closed-panel HMOs.

It is possible, however, for a psychologist to develop a single-service psychology HMO, which is essentially a prepaid mental health plan. Psychologist's should closely examine the state regulatory requirements for these entities; most HMO laws were drafted to accommodate only those entities offering full basic health services. State insurance regulators typically exercise broad discretionary power, so each state law must be examined separately. Most prepaid mental health plans have been developed to market a closed-panel capitated arrangement directly to a medically based, full-service HMO. The prepaid mental health plan "carves out" the mental health portion of the full-service HMO benefit package and assumes the responsibility for providing such services in exchange for a fixed prepaid fee from the HMO.

Some states (e.g., Texas, California, and Ohio) have enacted legislation that would regulate these prepaid entities. However, if there are no appropriate laws to regulate such entities, it appears that most states will permit a prepaid psychology plan to contract only directly with HMOs and not directly to the individual subscribers or employers. This stipulation is intended to protect subscribers. Because full-service HMOs and insurance companies maintain re-insurance, liability coverage, and reserves, if the single-service plan offers its services through an HMO, the subscribers can look to the full-service HMO for relief in the event that the single-service plan becomes insolvent. State regulators may be concerned that no such protection exists when single-service plans act as their own insurer.

Like HMOs, PPOs tend to be medically controlled, often sponsored by hospitals, medical IPAs, physicians, and insurance companies. Psychologists may find it difficult to achieve board membership or ownership unless they serve as an actual organizer or broker. Psychologist-owned and managed PPOs run into difficulty when purchasers want to negotiate a comprehensive mental health package that would entail providing inpatient care and medication management. Board equality between psychiatrists and psychologists is forbidden, as was mentioned earlier, by some state laws. Whereas a group of physicians can band together to form a PPO that can negotiate with area businesses to provide services, in many states physicians and psychologists cannot form a corporation together with the purpose of providing comprehensive mental health services. Some state laws prohibit members of different professions from forming a corporation together. For example, a group of psychologists attempted to incorporate with an IPA-model HMO in Illinois but were forced to incorporate as a separate IPA because state law prohibited their joining the medical IPA. Thus, state laws can sometimes serve to encumber psychologists' full participation in managed-care systems. Generally, individual state laws must be reviewed on a case-by-case basis to determine how each particular state law can be amended to minimize inappropriate barriers for psychological practice.

Ownership of an EAP entity that provides services to an organization as either a profit or a nonprofit vendor is possible for psychologists. In fact, social service and mental health agencies have entered the competitive EAP arena to increase their community base and resulting revenues. Probably the least cumbersome option for psychologists is to form a for-profit firm. Establishing an EAP firm as sole proprietor can be done as either an unincorporated business or a private corporation. Psychologists considering this option should seek financial and legal expertise to determine the appropriate choice and to file the required documents pursuant to state law. EAP ownership has advantages and disadvantages. On the positive side, owners have a great deal of control over how time can be spent, the selection of clients, and the quality of service. In contrast, owners must be concerned constantly about whether they have sufficient cash on hand to support ongoing marketing costs and to maintain overhead costs between initial proposal and final contract. When establishing a private EAP firm with colleagues, financial risk and decision-making are shared. Ownership requires a clear understanding of each partner's personality and well-developed techniques for resolving conflict. This is a marriage in which relationships among owners can greatly affect the firm's success.

Psychologists as Shareholders

Shareholders of managed-care entities stand to benefit financially as they would in any other stock investment. Psychologist-shareholders need to be aware of some dilemmas that may be posed by the potential for profit. By charter, managed-care entities are obligated to keep expenses down. Obviously, successful cost containment helps ensure a more positive return on investment for shareholders. Psychologist-shareholders have an ethical obligation to ensure that treatment decisions and quality of care are not compromised by cost factors. For example, cost containment should not be the sole justification for denying or curtailing treatment or for refusing to reimburse patients for outside referral (just as increasing profits should not be the sole justification for recommending more or more expensive treatment than is necessary). Similarly, psychologist-providers should be aware of their managed-care entity's hiring practices, specifically, the practice used by some staff-model HMOs of hiring lesser-qualified specialty providers as a means of controlling costs.

Shareholders of private EAP firms share financial risk, not responsibility. The degree of direct involvement can be individually determined and is flexible.

Psychologists as Independent Providers

Independent providers function as private practitioners who are reimbursed for their services either on a capitation or a reduced fee-for-service basis. In a capitation arrangement with an HMO, a financial agreement is made between the provider and the HMO, whereby the psychologist is paid monthly, based on specified cost factors and the number of members of the HMO that month. The issue of risk is a major concern in capitation arrangements. In awarding a capitation contract, the managed-care group is eliminating or reducing its financial risks for mental health services by passing them on to the provider. The provider agrees to provide mental health services to all of the covered (insured) members according to the HMO's limits. In theory, this means that, in an HMO with 50,000 members, the contracting provider has agreed to provide services for each and every member. In actual practice, however, only a small percentage of the members will utilize a provider's services, and, in established HMOs, this utilization rate remains fairly stable. Therefore, the risk is relatively small, especially if the provider is contracting only for outpatient mental health care. Contracting for comprehensive mental health services (i.e., outpatient, inpatient, and sometimes drug or alcohol treatment—inpatient and outpatient) significantly increases the risks, but again, the utilization of these services in established managed-care groups is fairly stable, and providers are given a reasonable projection of costs. Regardless of the range of services provided on a capitated basis, eventually professional and support staff will be needed. The capitation model characteristically necessitates allotting time for administration and other nonclinical responsibilities. Psychologists have considerable freedom as independent providers, and opportunities for financial growth considerably surpass those found for psychologist-employees of managed-care groups.

The managed-care group contracting out mental health services will establish with the psychologist or mental health group some agreement regarding an acceptable wait for nonemergency and emergency appointments. Arrangements will need to be made for on-call availability after hours and for hiring or contracting with psychiatrists or other professionals as the need arises. In addition, independent providers must follow local licensing and practice laws that govern who may be legally employed.

A variant of the independent provider is the subcontractor. A professional group or corporation that is responsible for providing mental health benefits may subcontract a special service (such as neuropsychological assessment) to specific providers, on a referral basis, for a specified price. Because the professional group or corporation that has the HMO contract for these mental health services is the gatekeeper, the subscriber has no direct access to the provider.

Psychologists can also be independent providers to an EAP. Psychologists, for example, working in this setting have more independence and less economic security than do their counterparts who are employed either directly by a business organization with its own EAP or with an EAP vendor who contracts with business organizations. Because EAPs usually provide only crisis intervention and brief counseling, they refer employees and family members who need more extensive treatment to community-based mental health professionals. The psychologist, in this position, has the primary relationship with the individual employee or family member rather than with the organization. The psychologist, therefore, has only one client—the individual. Because there is no contract, there is no guarantee of regular referrals. Independent providers can increase the likelihood of referrals by marketing themselves to EAPs.

Psychologists as Paid Employees

As employees of managed-care groups, psychologists may work in large, organized mental health departments with clearly defined guidelines. In smaller HMOs, however, the psychologist may be the sole provider of mental health services. Psychologist-employees of a managed-care group provide services within the benefit design limits similar in some ways to working within community mental health settings. The types of services provided vary with the size and type of group. In HMOs with smaller staffs, psychologists are more likely to be generalists, whereas in larger HMOs, specialized service models may prevail. Because service needs are typically high, volume considerations may prevail, and mental health providers may be expected to maintain high levels of clinical service, with few opportunities for research or training. Depending on the size of the HMO and state licensing laws, psychologists may also provide supervision, both for other psychologists and for nonpsychologists.

Some managed-care systems require patients to be seen by a physician prior to referral for mental health services, whereas others allow for self-referral by the patient. In either case, psychologists will interact routinely with other health care providers who may have limited understanding or appreciation of psychology. The opportunity to expand psychological knowledge is considerable when working with other health care providers in a collegial setting. A pediatrician who sees asthmatic children, for example, may call upon a psychologist to work with children who need to learn how to relax; a surgeon may ask a psychologist to render an opinion regarding the emotional stability of a patient being considered for open-heart surgery; and a nurse who is developing a weight-control or medication compliance program may seek input. These are typical of the requests psychologists may receive in such settings.

Opportunities for advancement within a staff-model HMO may be somewhat limited. As clinicians, psychologists may function in the more traditional roles of service providers, supervisors of therapists, psychology interns, and mental health administrators. Further advancement may require assuming more administrative responsibilities. HMO salaries vary by geographic areas and by employer, but they are typically lower for psychologist-employees than for psychologists who provide the same services on a fee-for-service basis. However, job security, benefits, and opportunity for professional growth are considerable in the staff-model HMO, and the overhead costs of private practice are not incurred.

Psychologists working in EAP settings can be employed in two ways. As a part- or full-time salaried employee working directly for the business organization that sponsors the managed-care entity, a psychologist may function as a mental health administrator or as a direct service provider. In these situations, the psychologist may have two clients: the individual employee and family members and the business organization. As employees in non-mental-health-oriented business organizations, psychologists are more subject to the political conflicts within the company than they are in any other role. Psychologists can also be involved in an EAP as part-time or full-time salaried employees of a firm, practice, or agency contracted to provide services to a managed-care entity. Psychologists can contract to deliver mental health services or other services, such as management consultation.

Essential Skills and Knowledge for Psychologists Working in Managed-Care Settings

Short-Term Therapy

Short-term therapy is the primary and, in some cases, only therapeutic approach used to deliver mental health services in managed-care settings. Managed-care psychologists are expected to quickly and accurately diagnose an individual's presenting problems and determine whether they will be responsive to brief treatment models. Furthermore, because most managed-care entities offer basically the same specified treatment terms, that is, a limited number of sessions for each member per membership year for nonchronic problems, psychologists are expected to work within those parameters.

Some HMOs do offer expanded mental health packages that eliminate criteria such as chronicity, prior treatment, and responsiveness to brief psychotherapy, but these packages are usually bought at a higher premium by the employer and require higher copayments by the patient. Even in cases of expanded mental health benefits, however, short-term therapy is usually the preferred treatment model, and managed-care groups are likely to prefer mental health professionals who will use the established treatment approach. For this reason, prior experience with brief therapy models and with crisis intervention may provide good practical preparation for psychologists working in managed-care groups.

Managed-care groups are sometimes criticized for limiting mental health visits to short-term intervention. However, it should be noted that HMO utilization rates parallel the national average of eight sessions per year that was found in other mental health agencies and the Civilian Health and Medical Program of the Uniformed Services. Nonetheless, certain conditions are not responsive to brief therapy models, and a blanket prohibition against treatment of so-called chronic mental health problems does not address the mental health needs of such patients.

Business Management

Because psychologists typically have little or no say in the financial or business affairs of a staff-model managed-care system, a business background is not really necessary. In other managed-care settings, however, business knowledge may be crucial.

Psychologists who contract with managed-care entities will need to attend to standard business practices of running an efficient, cost-effective operation, as well as being involved in hiring and supervising staff, delegating responsibility, and managing finances. Perhaps most important, psychologists need to be knowledgeable enough to enter into sound contracts. Contracts with managed-care groups are legal, binding agreements that hold the psychologist responsible for the provision of services as set forth in the contract. Contracts may stipulate the conditions for assuming financial and liability risks, particularly in the case of capitated arrangements. For example, a contract may stipulate that if utilization increases dramatically but membership does not, the contracting psychologist will have to provide additional services to the membership without receiving additional salary. Or a contract may contain a discontinuance clause that empowers the managed-care entity to dismiss a psychologist under certain conditions. Obviously, psychologists review agreements carefully before signing, and they should seek outside legal counsel as appropriate (see chapter 5).

Marketing

In order to establish or maintain a relationship with a managed-care group, psychologists must be prepared to market their professional services, including within the managed-care entity. Moreover, they should know how the managed-care group's marketing department represents psychological services, because the primary source of referrals is other managed-care providers and employers. Competition is keen in the limited mental health market, so managed-care groups may prefer packaged programs that meet their needs and service expectations at a competitive cost. Packages that include inexpensive, specialized services such as smoking-cessation or stress-management programs and parent-effectiveness workshops may, therefore, have great consumer appeal.

Marketing is particularly important for EAPs, which have to be attractive both to potential users and to the company's management. Marketing strategies differ for internal versus external EAP programs; interval EAPs rely primarily on educating their users by publicizing the EAPs' existence and usefulness to the eligible population, sustaining ongoing awareness of their programs, and motivating managers and employees to use programs both proactively and in problem situations. Keeping the program alive within a company means constantly educating senior management to its usefulness and informing them of its overall successes. Because marketing is a component of the political life of work organizations, good marketing skills are one of the tools necessary for survival within an organization. Marketing skills are probably even more important for external EAP vendors, who must constantly pursue new accounts in addition to educating existing client companies on new ways the EAP services can be utilized. Psychologists practicing in either internal or external EAP models need to have well-developed marketing skills, including knowing how to communicate, in a simple and practical manner, the ways in which EAPs can solve problems. They also need to understand the delicate balance between the need to keep the business marketplace aware of the available services and the need by potential customers to view professionals as being neither overly pushy nor benignly ineffective.

Case Management

Managed-care groups comprise many medical specialties. Because mental health referrals can come from a variety of sources, psychologists will want to establish a working rapport with as many of these professionals as possible. A patient who is experiencing panic attacks, for example, could be identified or evaluated by an internist, a cardiologist, or a neurologist, each of whom may have an opinion on diagnosis and appropriate treatment. These multiple opinions can be the source of either help or frustration to the patient. Opinions can be shared on an informal basis or at a more structured case review or treatment review conference. Such interaction can be highly stimulating for the psychologist and, ultimately, beneficial for the patient.

Staff-model managed-care groups are specifically designed in principle to encourage a multidisciplinary approach. In such settings the various medical specialists may be located at one site or at a small number of sites. When such settings encourage or require integration of treatment approaches, psychologists also may benefit by having a more comprehensive understanding of the patient. The integration may also spur medical practitioners to have a better understanding of the effects of emotions on patients' physical health and to learn more about how physical health influences the emotions.

Managed-care groups aim mental health services primarily at people experiencing nonemergency conditions that are amenable to short-term intervention. Most managed-care groups also have specific procedures and guidelines that both providers and subscribers must adhere to when addressing an emergency. Psychologist providers must be clear on the treatment parameters permitted by the system in such cases. In systems in which there is limited access to inpatient care, psychologists should carefully delineate their roles and responsibilities to avoid any liability for care rendered on an emergency basis or charges of patient abandonment (see chapter 5).

Some HMOs, especially staff models in which multiple medical services are offered in one facility, may prefer that emergency mental health patients who may be disruptive be seen in some other setting, such as the local hospital emergency room. It would be wise to plan for such an event in advance so that convenience and quality care can be provided. It may be possible, for example, to make an arrangement with a local community mental health center to serve as a backup for such emergencies. During off hours, the psychologist's office needs to arrange for on-call coverage.

Voluntary or involuntary admissions for emergency inpatient mental health treatment must adhere to local and state guidelines. Planning for such events includes knowing which hospitals accept managed-care members, children, drug or alcohol abusers or addicts, and so forth; whether the patient's plan covers inpatient care; and what alternatives to inpatient care are available and covered. In some instances, the system might allow a direct psychologist referral to a hospital, whereas other managed-care groups will require that an on-call physician approve the hospitalization.

It is important to become informed of all the established rules and procedures for such cases. Some managed-care groups will penalize providers who do not follow established rules for emergency cases. For example, there may exist a policy within an HMO regarding potentially disruptive patients coming onsite in a crisis. In addition, there are usually established procedures regarding written policies and guidelines for handling emergencies.

Records Management

In large managed-care entities, patients' records are likely to be handled by several different people. If central chart keeping is the standard, with no separate mental health record, a psychologist's records may be accessible to a variety of staff. Some may review the chart to ensure that a professional entry has been made. The chart may also be seen by others who will be providing treatment to the patient, by lab and support staff, and by any other number of personnel. Psychologists should be familiar with the in-house requirements and policies for record keeping before charting begins. In most instances, confidentiality depends on the integrity of colleagues.

In a decentralized system, mental health care records may best be kept by the psychologist, but accountability or billing arrangements will necessitate some sharing of information. As the insurer, an HMO will require reports from the psychologist-provider that detail which patients the provider sees, the reasons behind treatment, the duration of treatment, and whether treatment will be provided. Thus, guidelines regarding release of confidential information must be understood by the patient when seeking services. Also, the provider of services will need to clarify any ambiguities with the HMO regarding information it requires. Psychologists should also be aware of the American Psychological Association's current policy on record keeping (see American Psychological Association, 1992).

Benefit Limitations

HMOs traditionally establish a fixed maximum number of assessment or therapy sessions for subscribers. In addition, managed-care plans may exclude certain conditions or types of patients from coverage, including mental health problems of a chronic nature, problems perceived as not being responsive to brief psychotherapy, recurring psychological problems, marital or family therapy, psychological testing, vocational counseling, and court-requested or ordered forensic evaluation. Because of the high costs of inpatient mental health care, when managed-care systems offer it at all, they usually have their own, separately articulated criteria. And because cases requiring inpatient care may raise the risk of litigation, the criteria for exclusion may be well defined. It is important, therefore, that psychologists become familiar with the managed-care system's policies and limitations on inpatient care, preferably before encountering a case that may need such treatment.

When managed-care entities do deny treatment, they may employ some of the following criteria:

- In order to determine chronicity, the provider may conduct an extensive intake history to determine a patient's prior treatment experience. Treatment summaries may also be obtained from other mental health providers.
- If there has been no prior treatment, or if the history is not available, the provider may use the revised third edition of the *Diagnostic and Statistical Manual of Mental Disorders* (*DSM-III-R*; American Psychiatric Association, 1987) and psychological assessment results to arrive at a diagnosis. Certain conditions will be excluded from coverage if they are defined as chronic by the *DSM-III-R*.
- Chronicity may also be determined if the patient has been awarded Social Security benefits as a result of having emotional problems or is in any way diagnosed by some outside public agency as being disabled by emotional problems.
- Some managed-care entities, prior to denying services, may contract for a second opinion by an independent provider to evaluate the appropriateness of denial of service.
- Patients can also be denied services or have them curtailed if they are not compliant with treatment recommendations such as taking medication and keeping appointments. Denial of treatment for such reasons, however, may not legally protect an HMO if compliance is affected by the very nature of the patient's problem.

If patients are not excluded from treatment by these criteria, they must then pass the limitation based on "responsiveness to brief psychotherapy." This provision leaves considerable room for ambiguous interpretation in the absence of strictly defined criteria and a relevant research base. Psychologists who are responsible for deciding whether treatment is allowed are advised to be cautious about limiting mental health coverage solely on the basis of likelihood of short-term responsiveness. A decision to deny or limit care and its evidentiary rationale should carefully be documented. In such cases, the affected patient will often be informed in writing of his or her being denied treatment and of the rationale. Psychologists treating patients who have been denied coverage may need to determine their responsibilities, if any, for referral or ongoing treatment.

Utilization Review

Most managed-care systems have utilization review (UR) procedures. Because continued treatment can be denied on the basis of UR results, psychologists need to understand how such procedures work. Most UR committees base their decisions on statistical comparisons of the incidence and cost of treatment, by diagnosis and by provider. They look for statistical variance from the expected local or national norms. So, for example, if a psychologist-provider averages nine outpatient psychotherapy sessions per patient, and all other psychologists affiliated with the plan average six sessions, a UR committee might be concerned, especially if the provider is a persistent "outlier." The primary purpose of UR procedures is to ensure that services provided are valid, necessary, and appropriate. Scant empirical evidence exists, however, to suggest that the effectiveness of mental health care is enhanced by UR or cost containment (see chapter 9).

Utilization review committees are also usually responsible for the professional oversight of the managed-care entity's providers. Optimally, psychologists should be reviewed by psychologists, and separate peer review committees for psychological practice should exist. Indeed, psychologists should be allowed to sit on managed-care UR committees, as well as on peer review committees. The workings of one psychology peer review committee have been described by O'Keefe and Cress (1988).

In practice, however, UR committees are multidisciplinary and often medically controlled. Thus, psychologists frequently find themselves in the position of having to defend their mental health treatment decisions to physician gatekeepers or to members of other professions who may have the authority to overrule psychology-providers and deny or curtail psychological treatment. In order to defend their decisions and to ensure quality of care, psychologist-providers are often saddled with the burden of having to fill out complicated forms or write progress reports on a frequent basis. Some managed-care settings even require psychologists to justify continuation of care after each session.

Professional Roles and Relationships

Private practice psychologists are accustomed to assuming the role of independent practitioner. They function as sole proprietors or partners, with minimum confusion, in part because the roles are familiar ones. The role of employee of a mental health center, hospital, or HMO is also a known and comfortable one for many psychologist-practitioners. But, the emerging new forms of mental health delivery systems require that psychologists function in new and different ways, and in different roles. The role of entrepreneur is as confusing as it is potentially rewarding. The roles of investor, owner, and manager of a mental health delivery system are also new and available. Psychologists may not always know just how they fit in, what is expected of them, or even what is allowable. Such confusion is normal in a time of change and development.

For example, should psychologists who are members of an IPA-model PPO and who may, therefore, bid on contracts to provide psychological services, be prohibited from ever bidding for contracts as an individual psychologist or group-practice member? Psychologists need to clarify roles and rules before assuming their roles, and they need to identify, discuss, and work out possible solutions to potential conflict-of-interest issues in advance. Explicitly articulated policy in such situations is preferable. Ethical dilemmas can also arise. For example, if a preferred-provider psychologist or HMO staff psychologist determines that long-term therapy or some other noncovered benefit, such as marital counseling, is necessary, are self-referrals permissible? Or, what happens when an evaluating therapist, who is prohibited from self-referrals, is the locally recognized expert on problems such as those experienced by the client? Again, a clear-cut policy, explicitly communicated by the managed-care entity, may help to prevent potential problems.

Some psychologists now own or oversee capitated systems. They have a financial stake in treating patients as quickly and efficiently as possible. Each psychologist-provider will need to determine, on an individual basis, the balance between good patient care and cost efficiency. Especialy problematic are cases in which patients who begin brief therapy are found to need long-term therapy as facts of their psychological illness and background unfold. What are the psychologist's obligations when coverage, as it often does, runs out? Issues of patient abandonment and potential conflicts of interest need to be identified (see chapter 5 in this book).

Some potential problems will be specific to a particular managed-care setting. For example, does a psychologist who developed a test or wrote a book while in the employ of a staff-model HMO retain ownership rights to the test or book? Similarly, is a psychologist who is affiliated with an open-model HMO and who is known as the local expert in a particular field obliged to share his or her data or test results with other psychologists, even when it might cause personal financial loss? It will be some time before psychologists are comfortable with these new roles. In the meantime, common sense and collegiality may solve many problems as they arise.

The emergence of managed mental health care systems has apparently fueled another problem for psychologists: intraprofessional rivalry. Entrepreneurial skills have been highly rewarded in the managed-care arena. Some psychologists who saw the potential for financial gain early on, and who had the energy to pursue their vision, have done very well in the emerging mental health delivery systems. Others have not. This has been one source of misunderstanding and jealousy among psychologists.

Rivalry has also occurred on UR committees. Although most psychologists would probably agree that it is best to be reviewed by another psychologist, some psychologists sitting on UR or peer review committees have met with hostility from their colleagues when those colleagues were the subjects of reviews that were anything less than wholly positive. PPOs have also been known to contribute to intraprofessional problems. Because PPOs bid for contracts in competition with other PPOs and other psychologists, those excluded from the PPO and those not awarded the contract may be resentful. Moreover, when corporate managed-care entities control large amounts of the local mental health market, an exclusion may seriously affect a provider's income, if not be restrictive of trade and competition. Some psychologists employed by staff-model HMOs have reported hostility from psychology peers, who apparently view HMOs as being threatening to their practices and their professional security.

Interprofessional rivalry between psychologists and other health care professionals—most notably, physicians—has also increased with the emergence of managed care. The gatekeeper phenomenon that has been used in many managed-care systems appears to be one source of the problem. This practice, in effect, pits medical and psychology professionals against each other, by placing psychologists in the position of having their treatment decisions challenged by physicians who may, for example, value psychiatric intervention and medication more highly than psychological intervention or place more emphasis on cost containment or liability issues than on treatment issues. Furthermore, many HMOs and PPOs are owned and operated primarily by members of the medical profession. State laws that prohibit psychologists and psychiatrists from being partners in corporations can also be said to precipitate interprofessional problems and to block some of the easier solutions to these problems.

Liability

In today's litigious atmosphere, psychologists must be aware of liability issues and protect themselves as best they can. Any psychologist who works in association with another provider is potentially responsible not only for his or her own behavior but for that of the other providers as well. Generally, the closer the association, the greater is the liability. Anyone supervised or hired by the psychologist must, of course, have adequate skills, credentials, and, in the case of independent providers, sufficient malpractice insurance.

An emerging area of malpractice concern is that of patient abandonment. The potential for patient abandonment suits may be greater for alternative delivery systems such as HMOs and PPOs, which commonly end treatment early or after a few sessions as a means of controlling costs. For example, a managed-care UR committee may determine that a patient has received maximal benefits. The psychologist-provider and patient may not agree, but the managed-care entity still refuses to pay for the care, even after appeal. Psychologists in such cases must be careful not to be perceived as simply dropping the patient because benefits have run out and may have a duty to appeal the decision, to refer the case back to the managed-care group (or other source), or to continue treatment, at least temporarily, in order to avoid charges of patient abandonment (see chapters 5 and 7 in this book).

Psychologists should also make sure that they are legally protected in making decisions as members of managed-care UR committees. If a psychologist sitting on a UR committee goes along with a decision to curtail care and the patient sues the UR committee members for abandonment, would that psychologist be liable? Similarly, a psychologist who is involved as a preferred provider in a PPO could conceivably be one of the individuals sued under antitrust laws by a provider who is excluded from becoming a preferred provider of that PPO. The risk of being involved in antitrust legislation increases with level of involvement. A psychologist who is a board member, partner,

62   RESNICK ET AL.

shareholder, or owner of an HMO or PPO is at more risk than is a psychologist whose affiliation is solely as a provider.

Psychologists who are owners, partners, or board members of an IPA, PPO, or HMO could be sued as a result of malpractice or malfeasance on the part of a staff member, hospital, or provider with whom they contract; actions of the UR or quality assurance staff or committee members; violations of confidentiality; or even bodily injury suffered by a patient while traveling to the care facility. Any officer, owner, partner, or board member of an HMO or PPO must therefore have sufficient liability insurance coverage for any eventuality and to make sure credentials of contracting providers are carefully checked.

References

American Psychiatric Association. (1987). Diagnostic and statistical manual of mental disorders (3rd ed., rev.). Washington, DC: Author.
American Psychological Association, Board of Professional Affairs. (1992). Record keeping guidelines. Washington, DC: Author.
Health Maintenance Organization Act of 1973, section 280(c), 300(e)(1)(c)–(6)(a), 300(e)(1)(d), 300(e)(1)(b), 42 U.S.C. (1987).
O'Keefe, B. E., & Cress, J. N. (1988). Psychology peer review in an IPA-model HMO. In G. Stricker & A. R. Rodriguez (Eds.), Handbook of quality assurance in mental health (pp. 487–500). New York: Plenum.
Tax Equity and Fiscal Responsibility Act of 1982, Section 114(a), 42 U.S.C. [PL 97-248] (1986).

4

Parameters of Managed Mental Health Care: Legal, Ethical, and Professional Guidelines

Russ Newman
and Patricia M. Bricklin

Although some form of capitated health care has been in existence for many years, such as that sponsored by Kaiser Permanente, recently there has been a virtual explosion in alternatives to the traditional fee-for-service model of health care. *Managed care*, as it has become known, grew out of substantial changes in the economic realities of the health care marketplace in an attempt to contain the rising costs of health services.

Some people have argued that within the fee-for-service delivery system, health care was provided without regard to cost, and often without regard to necessity. This resulted in continued high costs of care during a period when the general economy was experiencing deflation. New cost-control and cost-reduction methods integrated into the service delivery system to prevent continued health care inflation have ultimately shaped the direction and spurred the growth of managed care. Enrollment in health maintenance organizations (HMOs), for example, grew 11.9% from December 1986 to September 1987, and included 28.8 million members. It is estimated that by 1993, 50 million people will be enrolled in HMOs nationwide (Martinson, 1988). This dramatic growth has been stimulated, in part, by legislation that removed some legal and financial obstacles to the creation of new managed-care entities.

Reaction to this change in the health care industry, particularly in the mental health care arena, has been mixed. A survey of psychologists and other mental health care professionals who subscribed to *Behavior Today* revealed that 86% of respondents believed that the quality of mental health care suffers when provided through managed-care structures ("BT Survey Results," July 20, 1987). The most frequent reason cited for the concern about quality in managed care was the limits or *caps* placed on the number of sessions a patient could receive—a complaint expressed by 79% of those surveyed. Other major complaints expressed included increased paperwork (67% of the respondents), the gatekeeping system (55%), decreased flexibility in the treatment ap-

Reprinted from *Professional Psychology: Research and Practice, 22*, 26–35. (1991). Copyright 1991 by the American Psychological Association.

proaches allowed (47%), and the long wait for reimbursements (46%); ("BT Survey Results," July 27, 1987). Approximately two thirds of respondents specifically objected to physicians and nurses with insufficient training and qualifications in mental health acting as gatekeepers.

Some advantages of managed health care were cited: increased client flow, less marketing needed by providers, added stability in an otherwise changing marketplace, and increased income–cash flow ("BT Survey Results," July 27, 1987). In general, the survey indicated that managed care was an economic benefit to providers at the expense of quality mental health care.

Perhaps the greatest focus of concern stimulated by managed care has been the potential adverse impact of financial incentives on the quality of care provided. Prepaid health care, the sine qua non of managed care, establishes a financial incentive to control costs. If the actual cost of treatment exceeds the prepaid amount, the managed care entity loses money. Therefore, it is in the best financial interest of the entity to provide no more treatment than the prepaid amount will support. Some fear this will lead to a treatment attitude focused on protecting some minimal level of care, in contrast to a fee-for-service treatment attitude of enhancing or maximizing the health of patients (Brook & Lohr, 1985). Furthermore, managed-care entities often give their participating providers financial incentives, such as bonuses, to hold down the actual cost of care rendered or arranged. Many are concerned that the incentives given to participating providers may be so strong that they pose a potential threat to the quality of care by encouraging inappropriate reduction in services (General Accounting Office [GAO], 1988). In fact, a recent study of depression found that patients receiving care financed by prepayment were significantly less likely to have their depression detected or treated than were similar patients receiving fee-for-service care (Wells et al., 1989). However, numerous mechanisms are potentially available within managed-care systems to provide parameters to counterbalance the potential adverse impact of cost-containment mechanisms and financial incentives. Strong management controls, such as quality assurance and utilization review, provider credentialing, medical records review, and enrollee satisfaction and grievance procedures, are necessary mechanisms to help identify and prevent provider behavior that adversely affects quality (GAO, 1988). Within an individual profession such as psychology, professional standards, ethical principles, and the risk of malpractice suits may also prevent behavior that adversely affects quality.

This chapter reviews the major legal (both legislative and common law), ethical, and professional parameters available to guide practitioners and managed-care entities in their endeavor to provide quality health care. Included among these parameters is a specific policy statement promulgated by the American Psychological Association (APA) that offers some recommendations to providers to minimize the potential for managed care's adverse impact on services.

Legislative Parameters

Federal Legislation

The earliest federal legislation to expressly address managed care was the Health Maintenance Organization Act of 1973 (HMO Act), which was enacted by Congress to facilitate the growth and development of HMOs around the country. Prior to the HMO Act, most state laws erected barriers to the creation of HMOs. In particular, many state laws classified HMOs as insurance companies, thereby requiring them to maintain considerable cash reserves as a condition of licensure. Although such cash reserves were readily available for traditional insurance companies, the requirement was often prohibitive for newly forming HMOs. The HMO Act preempted this type of state law requirement and, perhaps more important, made start-up funds available through a grant and loan program to new HMOs meeting broad standards.

Most of the requirements mandated by the HMO Act for an HMO to become federally qualified focus on financial and administrative arrangements. Included among these are the requirements of "a fiscally sound operation and adequate provision against the risk of insolvency" and assumption of "full financial risk on a prospective basis for the provision of basic health services." Only section 300(e)(7) of the HMO Act addresses quality-of-care concerns. It requires that an HMO "have organizational arrangements . . . for an ongoing quality assurance program for its health services which program (a) stresses health outcomes, and (b) provides review by physicians and other health professionals of the process followed in the provision of health services."

Mental health services required by the HMO Act (1973) are quite limited. Basic health services required by the act only include short-term outpatient evaluative and crisis intervention mental health services that cannot exceed 20 visits per year. Although basic health services include inpatient hospital services, the Code of Federal Regulations implementing the law considers inpatient mental health services to be *supplemental health services* that the HMO may provide but is not required to do. Most federally qualified HMOs, however, typically offer 30 inpatient days for mental health treatment as a part of their benefits. Required basic health services do include diagnosis, treatment, and detoxification for alcoholism or drug abuse on either an outpatient or inpatient basis, whichever is determined appropriate.

A second federally related boost to the managed-care industry was the Tax Equity and Fiscal Responsibility Act of 1982 (TEFRA). TEFRA provides for a managed-care alternative to Medicare's fee-for-service reimbursement system and enables Medicare to contract on a prepaid, fixed-cost basis (*risk contracts*) with selected HMOs to treat Medicare beneficiaries. Prior to TEFRA, few HMOs treated Medicare patients because the basic cost-containment mechanism of managed health care—prepaid, fixed-cost reimbursement—was unavailable. As of May 1988, approximately 1 million Medicare beneficiaries were enrolled in 137 HMOs (GAO, 1988).

It was not until 1986 that federal legislation began to include explicit restrictions on certain managed-care cost-containment strategies in order to address quality-of-care concerns. As a result of congressional concern that physicians may respond inappropriately to financial incentives, section 9312 of the Omnibus Budget Reconciliation Act of 1986 (OBRA) prohibits direct or indirect incentive payments by Medicare-participating hospitals to physicians to reduce or limit services. Furthermore, this section of OBRA prohibits HMOs with Medicare or Medicaid risk contracts from making incentive payments to providers. OBRA also mandates that care provided by TEFRA-created risk HMOs be monitored by peer review organizations (PROs) to prevent, or at least identify, abuses of care related to overly aggressive cost containment. The effective date for prohibiting HMO physician incentive payments, however, was subsequently extended to April 1, 1992, by the Budget Reconciliation Act of 1989. The apparent purpose of the extension was to allow sufficient time for Congress to study the actual potential of common financial incentive arrangements to inappropriately reduce or limit services.

At the time this chapter was written, one study by the GAO had concluded that the potential for financial incentive plans to threaten the quality of care provided is contingent upon the immediacy of the financial reward to individual treatment decisions and the extent of the risk transferred to providers (GAO, 1988). In other words, the closer in time the financial reward occurs to actual treatment decisions and the greater the amount of financial risk shifted from the HMO to the individual provider, the greater is the likelihood quality will suffer. Some HMOs, for example, pay providers a set fee with the expectation that it will cover services provided only by the primary provider; other HMOs pay providers a set fee and expect that it will cover primary provider care and specialist or hospital care as well in the event of referral. The latter arrangement places greater financial risk on the provider. The GAO has recommended that a ban on financial incentives be retained in situations in which financial reward is immediate and significant risk is shifted to the provider.

One piece of federal legislation that has a significant, albeit unintended, impact on care rendered by managed-care entities is the Employee Retirement Income Security Act of 1974 (ERISA). The net effect of various provisions in ERISA is that the federal law preempts state laws (i.e., state laws do not apply) for employee benefit plans, except to the extent that employee benefit plans otherwise involve activities that are regulated by state insurance law. Some employee benefit plans have argued that because of ERISA they need not comply with state-mandated benefits laws or provider laws (sometimes called *freedom-of-choice* laws). Thirty states statutorily mandate that insurance plans cover, or at least offer to beneficiaries a plan that covers, mental illness. Forty states mandate coverage for alcoholism, and 20 states mandate coverage for drug addiction. Forty-two states statutorily mandate that psychological services be covered by any plan that covers psychiatric services (National Center for Policy Analysis, 1988). Although the courts have narrowed the instances in which employee benefit plans are not subject to state mandates, ERISA preemption has reduced access to some mental health care.

In *Metropolitan Life Insurance Co. v. Massachusetts* (1985), the U.S. Supreme Court held that a state-mandated benefit law requiring certain mental health coverage was an insurance regulation and therefore was not preempted by ERISA when an employee benefit plan purchased insurance for its beneficiaries. This holding, however, did not apply to plans that did not purchase insurance and were self-insured (i.e., plans that themselves bear the risk of their beneficiaries' health costs). As a result, self-insured employee benefit plans can, if they wish, ignore state mandates and not cover mental health services or not offer freedom of choice of providers.

One limited exception to exemption from state law for self-insured plans occurs when the plan purchases *stop-loss* insurance from an insurance company. Stop-loss insurance assumes the risk of health costs when an aggregate ceiling of benefits is paid out by the self-insured plan. The United States Sixth Circuit Court, in *Michigan United Food and Commercial Workers Union v. Baerwaldt* (1985), ruled that a Michigan statute requiring all insurance policies to include substance abuse treatment coverage was not preempted by ERISA because the plan in question had purchased stop-loss insurance. In effect, the court held that a self-insured employee benefit plan was not truly self-insured when it purchased stop-loss insurance. In contrast to the Sixth Circuit holding, the Ninth Circuit ruled that a self-insured plan with stop-loss coverage was actually self-insured and exempt from state law (*Moore v. Provident Life and Accident Insurance Co.*, 1986).

Another exception to ERISA preemption of state law was articulated by *Northern Group Services v. Auto Owners Insurance Co.* (1987). The Sixth Circuit ruled that a coordination-of-benefits provision of the Michigan No-Fault Automobile Insurance Act was not preempted by ERISA in its application to self-insured plans. In arriving at this conclusion, the court reasoned that because the state's interest in a uniform administration of the no-fault insurance law outweighed any need for federal uniformity, the state law should not be preempted. It is important to note, however, that the court's holding was specifically based on the characteristics of the coordination-of-benefits provision of the no-fault automobile insurance law. As a result, the holding does not necessarily generalize to mandated benefits or freedom-of-choice laws.

The practical effect of ERISA preemption has been exclusion of coverage for psychological services by some self-insured employee benefit plans, many of which are structured as managed-care entities. Although most plans include some form of mental health and substance abuse coverage, a number of plans, (e.g., General Motors') have chosen not to cover the services provided by psychologists that would otherwise be required by freedom-of-choice laws.

It is possible that this exclusionary practice will be remedied by a court holding similar to that in *Northern Group Services v. Auto Owners Insurance Co.* (1987). A determination that state interests in uniformity outweigh a need for federal uniformity applied to freedom-of-choice laws could stop ERISA preemption. This is a difficult argument to make, however, because many of the employee benefit plans excluding psychologists are large enough to encompass employees in a number of states, thereby favoring an interest in federal, rather than state, uniformity. The most likely remedy would be passage of a federal law requiring national insurance coverage that expressly includes psychological services. Such a law would foreclose ERISA preemption for self-insured employee benefit plans.

State Legislation

All states regulate managed care to some degree in the form of HMO laws. All states require that HMOs be licensed at the state level. Furthermore, states have increasingly attempted to regulate the range of benefits offered, provider access, fiscal viability, and the quality of care provided. Because many HMOs have recently been withdrawing from the Medicare program—41 plans with a total enrollment of 87,000 subscribers dropped out in 1989 (National Health Lawyers Association, 1989)—fewer HMOs are federally qualified and subject to the federal preemption from state licensing laws that that status provides. State law is, therefore, becoming increasingly more important for regulation. Yet the degree to which HMO law actually regulates quality of care is quite limited.

In Massachusetts, for example, Chapter 176 G of the Annotated Laws of Massachusetts (1976) requires any health maintenance contract to provide for coverage of mental and nervous conditions and alcoholism. Section 8 of the Massachusetts statute regulates deceptive business practices and makes it illegal to disseminate "any promotional material, evidence of coverage in a health maintenance contract or any other statement with respect to a health maintenance organization which is untrue, deceptive or misleading." This provision addresses quality of care indirectly. In effect, an HMO must deliver services of the type and quality that it advertises being able to provide. An additional requirement for licensure, section 14(2), mandates that the HMO provide the commissioner of insurance with "a copy of the bylaws, rules and regulations, or similar documents regulating the conduct of internal affairs" of the HMO. No specific type or degree of internal regulation, however, is mandated.

The Model Health Maintenance Organization Act (Model Act) promulgated by the National Association of Insurance Commissioners (NAIC; 1989) recommends a model licensing law, which has been adopted in whole or in part by approximately one fourth of the states. It includes only very broad and general regulatory provisions. Section 4(a) (2) of the Model Act requires that an HMO applicant for licensure:

> (a) Has demonstrated the willingness and potential ability to assure that such healthcare services will be provided in a manner to assure both availability and accessibility of adequate personnel and facilities and in a manner enhancing availability, accessibility and continuity of service;
> (b) Has arrangements, established in accordance with regulations of the [commissioner of public health] for an ongoing quality assurance program concerning healthcare processes and outcomes; and
> (c) Has a procedure established in accordance with regulations of the [commissioner], to develop, compile, evaluate and report statistics relating cost of its operations, the pattern of utilization of its services, the availability and accessibility of its services, and such other matters as may be reasonably required by the [commissioner].

Clearly, much latitude is provided to the HMO to meet the statutory quality assurance requirements recommended by the model. The NAIC Model Act does, however, make specific reference to the potential adverse impact on quality of care of financial incentives in its "Comment" to subsection A(2):

> If the states are to authorize and encourage HMOs by this legislation, they have an obligation to assure that the healthcare services provided are of

reasonable quality. This is particularly true because of the built-in incentive for an HMO to restrict the utilization of services due to incentives to stay within a fixed budget.

The Model Act also establishes a system to provide reasonable procedures for enrollees to voice complaints about the care received. It further prohibits the use of untrue or misleading advertising or solicitation, and the use of deceptive evidence of coverage. Unfortunately, the Model Act expressly excludes mental health services or drug and alcohol abuse services from the basic health care services it recommends.

Other relevant state laws that have a bearing on parameters for managed care are mandated insurance benefits and mandated provider laws. In some states it is not entirely clear whether such laws apply to HMOs because HMO licensing laws have been promulgated separately and apart from preexisting insurance laws. Even in those states in which it has been determined that such preexisting insurance laws do apply to HMOs, confusion has been created by the more recent laws promulgated to specifically apply to HMOs. The statutory structure currently in place in Oregon exemplifies this confusion.

Section 743.123(i) of the Oregon Revised Statutes (1975) provides that health insurance subscribers "shall be free to select, and shall have direct access to, a psychologist . . . without supervision or referral by a physician or another health practitioner." This freedom-of-choice law has been determined to apply to HMOs, as well as traditional insurance indemnity plans. Section 743.556(23)(c) of the Oregon Revised Statutes (ORS 743.556), however, specifically allows HMOs to "limit the receipt of covered services by enrollees to services provided by or upon referral by providers associated with the health maintenance organization." Some HMOs have argued that the combinative effect of these two statutes requires them only to have a single psychologist on their panels of providers. If this is true, the practical effect of ORS 743.556 may be to negate freedom of choice and access by the HMO's subscribers to psychologists.

In an attempt to clarify the combinative effect of the two statutes, the Oregon Psychological Association (OPA) sued an HMO for its cost-containment practice of excessively limiting the number of psychologists on its provider panel (*OPA v. Physicians Association of Clackamas County*, 1989). In essence, OPA argued that the HMO's cost-containment procedures pursuant to ORS 743.556 were so excessive that they not only violated that law but also eviscerated the state's freedom-of-choice law. Although the case was recently dismissed by the Multnomah County Circuit Court, an appeal is currently pending in the Oregon Court of Appeals. The purpose of the appeal is to request the appellate court to determine at what point legally permissible cost-containment mechanisms become so extreme that they prevent statutorily required freedom of choice and access to psychological services.

Finally, state licensing laws for psychologists provide another potential mechanism for legislating parameters of practice in managed-care entities. A review of current licensing or certification laws in the 50 states and the District of Columbia revealed that none explicitly address the practice of psychology in managed-care settings (Bricklin, 1989). However, most state laws incorporate psychology's ethical principles. Therefore, to the extent that the profession's ethical code provides parameters for practice in managed-care settings (see the Ethical and Professional Practice Guidelines section), statutory parameters may also be established.

Parameters Created by Common Law

The shift in the health care marketplace toward managed care has modified or intensified legal issues present in the fee-for-service system and, therefore, has created a variety of new legal issues and potential liabilities (Elden, 1989). Without question, the potential for a managed-care entity and provider to be held liable for damages resulting from care given can have a profound effect on provider behavior. As a result, the development of new causes of action in the managed-care arena creates significant parameters for how care should be given.

Cost-Containment Liability

The first, and perhaps most revolutionary, case establishing new liability in managed care was *Wickline v. State of California* (1987; hereinafter referred to as *Wickline*). This case and its holding by the California Court of Appeals delineated the legal responsibility of a third-party payer for harm caused to a patient when a cost-containment mechanism is applied in a manner that affects the implementation of the provider's clinical judgment.

In *Wickline*, a MediCal (California's Medicaid program) beneficiary was hospitalized for an arteriosclerotic condition and underwent a surgical procedure to replace a portion of her artery with a synthetic graft. Because of complications, her physician requested from MediCal an 8-day extension to her originally preauthorized 10-day hospital stay. The MediCal utilization reviewer, however, authorized only a 4-day extension. As the patient's physician did not request any additional hospital days, she was discharged after a total of 14 days in the hospital. Subsequently, the patient developed a blood clot that necessitated the amputation of her right leg. The patient sued the state of California, alleging that MediCal's refusal to grant the additional 4-day extension caused her injuries. The trial court held for the plaintiff and awarded $500,000 in damages and found the utilization reviewer negligent.

The appellate court, however, reversed the verdict and found that MediCal was not liable for the patient's injuries. The court's reasoning was two-fold. First, because the treating physician did not protest MediCal's denial of the 8-day extension, MediCal was viewed as never having had the opportunity to override the physician's decision. Second, because it was concluded by the court that the blood clot and amputation would have likely occurred even if the patient had remained in the hospital another 4 days, MediCal could not be liable.

The court continued on, however, to discuss those situations in which third-party payers could be held liable for denial of care:

Third party payors of healthcare services can be held legally accountable when medically inappropriate decisions result from deficits in the design or implementation of cost-containment mechanisms as, for example, when appeals made on a patient's behalf for medical or hospital care are arbitrarily ignored or unreasonably disregarded or overridden. (*Wickline*, p. 1645)

The result, then, is that insurers, HMOs, other managed-care entities that act as third-party payers, employers, and utilization reviewers may be liable for harm when defects in cost-containment procedures, such as utilization review, lead to patient injury. These entities must now conduct themselves with this potential liability in mind.

Perhaps more relevant for psychologist-providers is the portion of the *Wickline* holding that a prospective denial of coverage may be viewed as a denial of care if the provider adheres to the payer's recommendation, *but only if the provider has first protested the payer's recommendation for length of treatment.* In effect, the psychologist must actively object to a utilization review decision if it is at odds with the psychologist's clinical judgment. However, in a recent California Court of Appeals decision, *Wilson v. Blue Cross of Southern California* (1990), the court held that the provider need not protest the utilization review decision to trigger potential liability on the part of the utilization review entity. In any case, it is important to note that the psychologist will not totally avoid treatment responsibility for the patient. Rather, both the treating provider and the utilization reviewer will share responsibility for premature termination of treatment.

Gatekeeping and Financial Incentives

Since *Wickline*, plaintiffs have utilized the case's precedent-setting theory of liability for cost-containment mechanisms to challenge managed-care entities' use of gatekeepers and financial incentives to limit medical care. (At the time this chapter was written, no such case involving mental health services had been filed. Yet it may be anticipated that if these challenges to medical care, where damages are more obvious, are successful, similar challenges involving mental health treatment will follow.) In *Bush v. Dake* (1987; Clerk of the Court, Saginaw County Court of Michigan, personal communication, April, 1990), a suit against a Blue Cross/Blue Shield-operated HMO in the Saginaw County Court in Michigan, the plaintiff charged that her cervical cancer was exacerbated by the failure of the HMO's primary physician gatekeeper to refer her to a specialist in time. Following a judicial ruling that a jury should decide whether the financial incentives contributed to the plaintiff's injury, the suit was immediately settled out of court with an agreement that prevents any of the participants from discussing the case.

Similarly, in *Sweede v. CIGNA Healthplan of Delaware* (1988), an HMO was being sued for its negligent use of a gatekeeping mechanism and financial incentives. The plaintiff, a woman with breast cancer, alleged that as a member of the CIGNA HMO, she was not referred to a specialist for more than a year after she visited her primary care physician and complained of a lump in her breast. She further alleged that by the time a referral was made, the cancer was inoperable. In addition, she argued that CIGNA used financial incentives to restrain its primary care physicians from using health care resources to treat CIGNA members. It is specifically alleged that these financial incentives create an inherent conflict of interest that may inappropriately influence provider behavior and adversely affect the quality of members' care.

The CIGNA plan subject to the lawsuit withholds 20% of all capitation fees earned by primary care physicians and 20% of all fees earned by participating specialists who treat members. These withholdings are retained in a *performance risk pool* subject to disbursement at the end of a 12-month period. If the actual cost of health care to its members exceeds CIGNA's budget, this 20% withholding is applied first to over-budget institutional service expenses (e.g., inpatient hospital care and emergency care) and second to over-budget professional and ancillary service expenses (e.g., surgeon's care). If the primary physician's entire 20% withholding is applied to cover expenses that exceed members' actual payments, then the participating physician forfeits this fee. This incentive system, according to the lawsuit, is designed to offer participating providers a financial incentive not to refer members for institutional, emergency, professional, and ancillary services. In effect, the court will decide whether care provided by CIGNA and its primary care physicians is compromised by financial incentives, and therefore is negligent.

Because none of these lawsuits that relate to the effect of gatekeeping and financial incentives had come to trial at the time this chapter was written, it is unclear how the courts may have decided these issues. The impact of these lawsuits on provider behavior, however, must still be considered significant. Providers cannot completely ignore the potential that practices currently accepted in the managed-care arena will eventually be deemed negligent by the common law, thereby subjecting these providers to legal and financial liability.

Disclosure of Financial Incentive Plans

The *Sweede v. CIGNA* case also alleges fraud and deceit by CIGNA because of its failure to disclose the financial incentive plan to prospective members. Specifically, the complaint alleges that CIGNA engaged in deceptive trade practices in violation of Delaware law by failing to inform consumers that its health care service used financial incentives to restrain providers from referring members to health care resources. It also complains that CIGNA created a likelihood of confusion that consumers were to receive the same quality health care as in a fee-for-service plan. This pattern of deceptive trade practices, according to the plaintiff, prevented her from making an informed decision whether to enroll in CIGNA's HMO or to remain in her fee-for-service plan. It is further charged that CIGNA acted in bad faith and breached its promise to refer the plaintiff to a specialist when necessary.

The most recent challenge to what has been considered common practice in managed care is *Teti v. U.S. Healthcare, Inc.* (1989), a class action suit brought in federal court in the Eastern District of Pennsylvania. In contrast to previous lawsuits, this action is not based on any allegation that plaintiffs have suffered any physical injury or that malpractice has occurred. Rather, the suit charges that U.S. Healthcare and its wholly owned subsidiary HMOs have violated the Racketeer Influenced and Corrupt Organizations Act of 1970 (RICO) and Pennsylvania's Unfair Trade Practices and Consumer Protection Statute, and have engaged in common-law intentional misrepresentation, fraud, and breach of contract.

The complaint focuses on the HMO's alleged failure to disclose to prospective members and actual subscribers the existence and nature of a financial incentive arrangement. This arrangement includes an incentive whereby primary physicians' compensation is reduced in proportion to the costs of their referral to specialists and inpatient hospital facilities. The suit claims that the HMO's promotional efforts, which advertise full coverage of hospital and specialist services but fail to disclose the financial incentive involved in the referral process, constitute a systematic and continuous scheme to mislead consumers and to misrepresent and conceal the true nature of the services available to members. These promotional efforts through the interstate mail and the failure to disclose financial incentive arrangements, according to the complaint, constitute a pattern of racketeering activity in violation of RICO.

Although the *Teti v. U.S. Healthcare, Inc.*, case was recently dismissed by the federal court because of its failure to satisfy some of the technical legal requirements of RICO, the claims of violation of Pennsylvania law and common law remain viable. It is likely that the case will be refiled in the state court that has jurisdiction over these remaining issues.

Credentialing Liability

To the extent that concerns exist regarding unqualified personnel providing treatment and gatekeeping functions in managed-care entities, potential liability for negligent provider selection by an entity may provide a useful parameter. In particular, the corporate negligence doctrine used to hold hospitals liable for negligent selection and supervision of personnel may be used to hold managed-care entities similarly accountable.

In *Darling v. Charleston Community Memorial Hospital* (1965), the Illinois Supreme Court held that a hospital owed an independent duty of care to the patient separate from the duty owed by the treating provider. This duty, said the court, was breached by the defendant-hospital failing to require examination of the plaintiff-patient by a qualified member of the hospital's staff. More to the point, the Georgia Supreme Court, in *Joiner v. Mitchell County Hospital Authority* (1971), held that if a physician's incompetence results in patient injury and the hospital knew or should have known of the physician's incompetence, the hospital is negligent for allowing the physician to become a member of its staff.

Numerous other cases have held hospitals liable for not providing proper overall supervision of the quality of care, for failing to properly review and investigate the credentials and expertise of medical staff applicants, and for failing to protect patients from malpractice by members of the medical staff when they knew or should have known that such malpractice was likely.

Although managed-care entities do not have custody of the patient in the same manner as do hospitals, provider selection by the entity, combined with the limitation or restriction of the patient's choice of providers, may create similar duties for managed-care entities (Elden, 1989). In fact, the corporate negligence doctrine was used to sue an HMO in *Harrell v. Total Healthcare, Inc.* (1988), but a Missouri trial court declined to rule on the merits and dismissed the case on procedural grounds. The Missouri Court of Appeals, however, sustained a motion for a rehearing and withdrew the trial court opinion. Thus, at the time this chapter was written, the case was still pending.

Ethical and Professional Practice Guidelines

Given the relatively limited statutory controls on the use of cost-containment mechanisms within managed-care entities and the potential for provider liability, it is incumbent upon individual providers to balance quality with cost containment. In fact, the effect of incentive arrangements on good providers are believed to be distinguishable from the effects on bad providers (ICF, 1987). More specifically, the result of incentives for good providers is likely to be cost-effective quality care, whereas the result for bad providers is likely to be inexpensive but poor care. This is perhaps not unlike the result of financial concerns in a traditional fee-for-service model of health care. In other words, it may be speculated that some providers may take advantage of lucrative insurance funds by extending care beyond what is medically or psychologically necessary.

It is difficult, if not impossible, to screen out those providers who will sacrifice quality for financial rewards, but appropriate ethical parameters for provider behavior can minimize such abuses. Some guidance for psychologists working in managed-care settings can be found in the *Ethical Principles of Psychologists* (APA, 1990), although none of these principles expressly refers to psychological services in managed-care settings.

Principle 1(f), pertaining to responsibility, mandates that psychologists as practitioners be "alert to personal, social, and organizational, financial, or political situations and pressures that might lead to misuse of their influence" (p. 633). Every psychologist must be cognizant of the organizational structure of managed-care entities focused on cost containment and the related financial pressures. More to the point, psychologists are ethically bound to take care that these pressures not result in treatment that is to the detriment of patients.

In addition, Principle 6 (welfare of the consumer) provides that "when conflicts of interest arise between clients and psychologists' employing institution, psychologists clarify the nature and direction of their loyalties and responsibilities and keep all parties informed of their commitments" (p. 636). This principle may be construed to resolve any conflict arising between a managed-care entity (or provider's financial interest) and quality of care concerns in favor of the latter. At the very least, the principle argues for disclosure to the client that a financial incentive exists to keep the amount or type of service limited.

Although not proscriptive in the same way as the *Ethical Principles*, the *General Guidelines for Providers of Psychological Services* (*Guidelines*; APA, 1987) may delineate parameters of behavior within managed-care settings. In fact, the *Guidelines* are intended to apply to psychological services "at any time and *in any setting* [italics added]" for the purpose of promoting the "best interests and the welfare of users of such service" (p. 1). Furthermore, the preamble recognizes that principles of conduct "evolve over the history of every profession . . . [which] guide the relationships of the members of the profession to their users, to each other, and to the community of which both professional and users are members" (p. 1). Yet few of the actual guidelines appear relevant to the unique concerns of managed care's cost-containment emphasis.

Only Guideline 3 (accountability) has some relevance to the dilemma created for psychologists by the competing concerns of cost containment and quality of care. In particular, Guideline 3.1 indicates that "the promotion of human welfare is the primary principle guiding the professional activities of all members of the psychological service unit" (p. 7). A plausible interpretation of this guideline is, in effect, that cost containment stops where quality of care begins to be compromised. The illustrative statement intended to clarify this guideline expressly prohibits the withholding of services to a potential user. Unfortunately, the influences listed as potential causes of withholding of services—national or ethnic origin, religion, gender, affectional orientation, or age—indicate that the *Guidelines* did not envision the possibility of services being withheld because of financial incentives or cost-containment concerns.

Guideline 2.3.4 is of similar indirect relevance to the unique situation created by managed-care structures, particularly the situation of disclosure of a provider's financial incentives to consumers. That guideline states, "Professional psychologists clarify early on to users and sanctioners the exact fee structure or financial arrangements and payment schedule when providing services for a fee," (APA, 1987, p. 6). Unfortunately, the illustrative statement speaks only to traditional fee-for-service reimbursement procedures.

In addition, Guideline 3.4 makes professional psychologists accountable for all aspects of the service they provide, including financial concerns. The illustrative statement indicates that this accountability includes the provision of accurate and full information to the user regarding the qualifications of providers, the nature and extent of services offered, and, where appropriate, financial costs and potential risks.

Although the ideal incorporated by this guideline is laudable and relevant to managed care, the feasibility of its implementation may be questionable. If a psychologist is held accountable for all aspects of his or her services provided within a managed-care structure, the result may be individual accountability for aspects over which the psychologist has no control. For example, should a psychologist-provider employed by a managed-care entity be held accountable for corporate policies that emphasize the financial bottom line or implement financial incentives to the point that quality of care suffers? Or should the psychologist-provider be held accountable for the corporation's advertising that does not thoroughly describe the financial incentives inherent in managed care to reduce the amount or type of treatment it provides? Taken to its logical extreme, this guideline might make it impossible for psychologists to work within some managed-care settings. Whether one agrees with this result or not, it is unlikely that such an outcome was envisioned by the drafters of the *Guidelines.*

APA Policy on Managed Care

Although some legislative, ethical, professional, and common law parameters for providing treatment within managed care settings do exist, they are considered by many in organized psychology to be either slow in developing or insufficient to deal with the unique characteristics of the newly emerging health care system. As a result, the APA's Council of Representatives promulgated a policy statement in 1988 designed to articulate organized psychology's concerns about the potential effects of managed care on psychological services. Furthermore, the policy was intended to offer some recommendations to providers and consumers, in an attempt to minimize the potential for managed care's adverse effects on services (APA, Council of Representatives, 1989). Since that time, APA boards and committees have taken various steps to implement the spirit of the council policy statement, which remains as APA policy to the present.

Background and Policy Development

In the early 1980s, as a result of activities at the federal level and the emergence of new alternative health care delivery models, many psychologists in practice approached the APA through individual letters expressing interest and concern about these new service delivery systems. In response, APA, through its Board of Professional Affairs (BPA), began to explore managed care in the context of future markets for psychological practice. At that time, there was both a growing excitement about the possibility of managed care as a creative solution to service delivery problems and a concern about the possible legal and ethical issues presented by such an alternative model.

Between 1982 and 1984, BPA sponsored a major APA convention program to review the issues and, as a result, established a Subcommittee on Future Markets. While developing a manual for providers interested in preferred provider organizations (PPOs), HMOs, and other managed-care models, the Subcommittee on Future Markets considered issues of helping psychologists cope with the other emerging cost-containment measures, the need for peer review in the system, and especially the need to educate providers on both the negative and positive aspects of involvement in alternative delivery systems. Despite these efforts to educate the APA membership about the changing health care marketplace, by 1985 it was clear that changes and events in this arena were occurring more rapidly than had been anticipated. These changes had serious ramifications for the delivery of psychological services, as evidenced by the growing concern expressed by state associations, divisions of APA, and individuals (APA, Committee for the Advancement of Professional Practice, 1988). In addition, other APA governance groups associated with public interest expressed particular concern over access-to-care and quality-of-care needs of special populations within these systems.

In response, the BPA approved the development of a manual to educate the APA membership about the opportunities and challenges facing psychologists interested in joining HMOs and PPOs. The manual, *Marketing Psychological Services: A Practitioner's Guide* (APA, 1986), was completed in late 1985 and published in 1986.

During the same period, the APA Committee on Women in Psychology, the Committee on Gay and Lesbian Concerns, and the Board of Social and Ethical Responsibility reviewed managed-care issues with respect to care and quality-of-care needs of special populations within managed-care systems. As a result of their deliberation, they expressed the following concerns:

1. As the primary aim of new service delivery systems is cost containment, comprehensiveness of service or provision for services for special populations or special needs may not be specified.

2. There are serious problems with preferred provider organizations and other newly emerging health care delivery systems which, because of a lack of built-in regulatory mechanisms, do not ensure consumer access to a diversity of providers. This is an issue of particular importance for gay and lesbian clients, ethnic minority populations, and women.

3. The new models of health care delivery are not bound by regulations that would require psychologists, especially those who specialize in working with specific populations (i.e., women, ethnic minorities, lesbians and gays, older persons), to be included. As a result, there is a strong probability that women and other special populations will have to accept less than optimal services or pay for psychotherapy outside their health plans (APA, Committee on Gay and Lesbian Concerns, 1984, p. 6; APA, Board of Social and Ethical Responsibilities, 1984 p. 5; APA, Committee on Women in Psychology, 1985, p. 11).

4. Regarding HMOs, there are four areas of particular concern: training of personnel to deal with minority populations; quality assurance with ethnic minority populations; truth-in-packaging issues; and the need for legislation that affects ethnic minorities (APA, Board of Ethnic and Minority Affairs, 1986).

The particular concern for public interest groups, especially those that work with minority populations, is that the majority of managed-care systems designate care providers. In a managed-care model, the patient generally has the choice only of providers who are part of the system. These providers may or may not be sensitive to minority issues. In a really free enterprise system, the client is free to choose a provider who is sensitive to his or her specific minority concerns. It is critically important that clients who enter into managed-care systems be aware that they may be limited in their choice of service provider. This is a real truth-in-packaging issue.

The issue of psychologists' participation in alternative managed health care delivery systems continued to be of concern to various APA groups, including public interest and practice-oriented constituencies. With the creation of the Office of Professional Practice within APA, its Interim Advisory Committee became a coordinating mechanism for consideration of managed care.

The Interim Advisory Committee (later Committee for the Advancement of Professional Practice) expressed concern over additional issues in managed care in 1988 (APA, Interim Advisory Committee, 1988). The concern that cost containment would be the chief driving force in treatment decisions at the expense of the consumer was a major issue. It affirmed that it is especially important that decisions regarding quantity and quality of care be based on consumers' needs, as well as on the economic interest of the health care delivery system. A proposed policy statement developed by the Interim Advisory Committee was circulated to all interested APA governance groups, including the BPA, and appropriate public interest groups, including the Committee on Women in Psychology and the Committee on Gay and Lesbian Concerns (APA, Committee for the Advancement of Professional Practice, 1988). This culminated in a document unanimously agreed upon by all of the participating groups, which was presented to the Council of Representatives in August 1988 and became APA policy at that time.

Policy Statement by the Council of Representatives

WHEREAS, many mental health problems are reflective of profound problems of living, substantial intra-psychic disorganization or severe physical and psychological disruption; and

WHEREAS, some psychological services are specifically focused on the alleviation of the personal distress attendant thereto; and

WHEREAS, managed care or other health care delivery systems should not unduly discriminate against those consumers who need intensive care, against those who need specialty care, and should not systematically endorse short-term or biomedical intervention as the treatment of choice for all patients at the expense of individual needs; and

WHEREAS, managed care delivery programs, by their very nature, frequently impose artificial and/or economic barriers to consumer access to health care services and, as such, are as subject to mismanagement as are traditional funding and delivery systems; and

WHEREAS, many managed health care programs may unfairly exclude those with the greatest need from adequate care and/or otherwise put both consumer and participating professional at substantial economic/psychological risk; and

WHEREAS, it is important that mental health care delivery programs provide appropriate and equally high quality services to all persons in diverse client and underserved populations; and

WHEREAS, providers and patients should be informed of the limitations and restrictions to types and access of psychological services prior to subscribing to a plan (i.e., truth in advertising or explicit statements regarding any financial disincentives to treat and refer patients in need of psychological services),

THEREFORE, BE IT RESOLVED that the American Psychological Association urges consumers, subscribers and psychologists to review carefully the mechanisms, procedures, practices and policies of managed care programs before deciding to participate. Although such programs may offer the potential to expand access to appropriate mental health care, they may also restrict the availability of necessary psychological services.

It is further recommended that providers may wish to require as a condition of their participation that such managed health care delivery systems adequately and concretely demonstrate provisions to serve the consumer's interest with sufficient quantity and highest quality of health care based on the available scientific evidence of efficacy.

It is further recommended that consumers, subscribers and psychologists, as a condition of their participation, require that these programs practice truth in advertising regarding the range and duration of psychological services available through the plan and that these programs provide patients access to diversity of psychological health care competencies based on the available scientific evidence of efficacy.

It is also recommended that providers require that such systems operate in accordance with prevailing standards of care and prevailing scientific knowledge, applicable ethical principles, and that the systems have sufficient economic resources to cover the delivery system's liability.

Finally, individual members, state psychological associations and divisions are strongly urged to monitor and inform themselves of the legal and regulatory requirements imposed on managed health care systems and to advocate that such requirements meet the principles enumerated herein. (APA, Council of Representatives, 1989, p. 1024)

This alternative health care delivery policy continues to be APA policy into the 1990s. Since its passage, APA has initiated a number of activities to implement the policy. Specifically, APA, through its boards and committees, has initiated the following implementation steps:

1. Communication of the APA Council of Representatives policy and its advisory statements to state associations.

2. The development of a manual on alternative health care delivery systems, to be distributed to psychologists in professional practice.

3. Active lobbying on the part of the Practice Directorate of the American Psychological Association for HMO and PPO legislation to protect consumers and members.

The APA is not the only professional mental health provider group expressing concerns about the potential effects of managed care on mental health services. The American Psychiatric Association Board of Trustees recently created the Ad Hoc Committee on Managed Care Issues and voted to earmark up to $50,000 to investigate legal issues and concerns about managed care

(American Psychiatric Association, 1990). The board also voted to support the concept of developing acceptable practice parameters for psychiatric care.

Conclusions and Recommendations

The most significant component of managed care, and that which has raised concerns among psychologists and other health care providers, is its focus on cost containment. Strategies implemented to reduce health care costs do not, per se, result in poor quality care. However, the potential for an adverse impact on the quality of care provided within managed-care entities is a reality that must be dealt with, particularly when cost-containment strategies such as financial incentives for providers are taken to an extreme.

Some legislative, common law, ethical, and professional parameters do exist in order to help psychologists draw the line between cost-effective, quality care and compromised care. Yet, the basic tension between cost containment and quality care continues to create ambiguity for providers accustomed to providing treatment in a traditional fee-for-service model. In particular, ethical and professional guidelines for psychologists have been developed with little direct attention to the unique issues raised by managed care. Although some degree of accountability for treatment provided by and within managed-care entities is, or threatens to be, imposed by common law, after-the-fact imposition of liability is hardly an ideal way to ensure good care.

It is incumbent upon organized psychology to develop clearer guidelines for the provision of services in the managed-care setting. The policy statement promulgated by the APA may be helpful, although such a statement cannot be expected to have the same impact on psychologists as proscriptive ethical principles or even aspirational professional guidelines. It is recommended that the existing *Ethical Principles* and *General Guidelines* be amended to reflect the potential impact of cost-containment strategies on psychological services. Conceptually, such principles or guidelines should underscore the importance of maintaining quality care in the fact of managed-care cost-containment strategies, rather than attempt to specifically direct the provision of psychological services.

It is also necessary for psychology to influence the development of clearer legislative and legal parameters for mental health services provided in the managed-care arena. This can be accomplished by advocacy efforts such as those currently being planned by the APA's Practice Directorate. Federal and state legislation should be enacted to require HMOs to expand services by increasing available benefits and to require continuation of benefits for patients who exhaust the limited number of sessions when additional treatment is necessary. Laws that prohibit financial incentive arrangements from sacrificing quality care and that establish better quality-control mechanisms must be actively advocated. In addition, utilization review mechanisms must be strengthened by legislation so that they actually distinguish between necessary and unnecessary care and are not used simply to reduce the amount of treatment in the service of cost savings.

Lawsuits that help to clarify existing legal parameters and establish common-law accountability should be encouraged, if not initiated. Managed-care entities that promote financial interests to the detriment of patient care should be held responsible for any adverse impact on patients.

Perhaps above all, psychologists have an obligation to help educate consumers about the potential benefits and problems inherent in mental health services rendered through managed-care entities. The research methods and critical self-examination characteristic of psychology must be applied to managed care to sort out effective from adverse treatment consequences. Only then can consumers make a truly informed choice about the care they wish to receive.

References

American Psychiatric Association. (1990, January 5). Trustees attack managed care treat. *Psychiatric News*, p. 1.

American Psychological Association. (1986). *Marketing psychological services: A practitioner's guide*. Washington, DC: Author.

American Psychological Association. (1987). *General guidelines for providers of psychological services*. Washington, DC: American Psychological Association, Committee on Professional Standards.

American Psychological Association. (1990). Ethical principles of psychologists (amended June 2, 1989). *American Psychologist, 45*, 390–395.

American Psychological Association, Board of Ethnic and Minority Affairs. (1986, May 1–3). *Minutes*. Washington, DC: American Psychological Association, Public Interest Directorate.

American Psychological Association, Board of Social and Ethical Responsibilities. (1984, November 2–4). *Minutes*. Washington, DC: American Psychological Association, Public Interest Directorate.

American Psychological Association, Committee for the Advancement of Professional Practice. (1988, March 18–20). *Exhibit 1, Summary Board of Professional Affairs actions related to alternative healthcare delivery systems*. Washington, DC: American Psychological Association, Practice Directorate.

American Psychological Association, Committee on Gay and Lesbian Concerns. (1984, September 28–29). *Minutes*. Washington DC: American Psychological Association, Public Interest Directorate.

American Psychological Association, Committee on Women in Psychology. (1985, March 28–30). *Minutes*. Washington, DC: American Psychological Association, Public Interest Directorate.

American Psychological Association, Council of Representatives. (1989). Proceedings of the American Psychological Association, Incorporated, for the year 1988. *American Psychologist, 44*, 996–1028.

American Psychological Association, Interim Advisory Committee. (1988, January 8–10). *Managed care systems*. Washington, DC: American Psychological Association, Practice Directorate.

Annotated Laws of Massachusetts. (1976). 176-G Mass. Anno. Laws § 47(B), St. Paul, MN: West.

Bricklin, P. (1989, January). *Licensing boards and supervision*. Paper presented at the American Psychological Association of State Psychology Boards, midwinter meeting, New Orleans, LA.

Brook, R., & Lohr, K. N. (1985, May). Efficacy, effectiveness, variations, and quality: Boundary-crossing research. *Medical Care*, 720–722.

BT survey results: The changing mental healthcare delivery system. (1987, July 20). *Behavior Today*, 1–2.

BT survey results: Advantages and disadvantages of HMOs. (1987, July 27). *Behavior Today*; 1–2.

Budget Reconciliation Act of 1986, 42 U.S.C. §§ 280, 300(e)1(c)–(6)(a), 300(e)(1)(d), 300(e)(1)(b).

Budget Reconciliation Act of 1989 (PL 101-239, December 19, 1989). *Code of Federal Regulations.* (1987, October). 42 C.F.R. §§ 417.10(a)(b). St. Paul, MN: West.

Darling v. Charleston Community Memorial Hospital, 211 N.E. 2d 253(1965).

Elden, D. (1989, June). *Managed care legal issues.* Paper presented at the 1989 Health Law Update, National Health Lawyers Association, San Francisco, CA.

Employee Retirement Income Security Act of 1974, 29 U.S.C. § 1142 (1982).

General Accounting Office. (1988). *Medicare physician incentive payment by prepaid health plans could lower quality of care* (GAO/HRD-89-29). Washington, DC: U.S. Government Printing Office.

Harrell v. Total Healthcare, Inc., Missouri Court of Appeals, West District (1988).

Health Maintenance Organization Act of 1973, 42 U.S.C. §§ 280(c), 300(e) (1)(c)–(6)(a), 300(e)(1)(d), 300(e)(1)(b). (1987).

ICF. (1987). *Physician incentive arrangements used by HMOs and PPOs* (Report submitted to the Office of the Assistant Secretary for Planning and Evaluation, DHHS). Washington, DC: U.S. Government Printing Office.

Joiner v. Mitchell County Hospital Authority, 186 S.E. 2d 307 (1971).

Martinson, J. N. (1988). Are HMOs slamming the door on psychological treatment? *Hospitals, 62,* 50–56.

Metropolitan Life Insurance Co. v. Massachusetts, 471 U.S. 724 (1985).

Michigan United Food and Commercial Workers Union v. Baerwaldt, 767 F. 2d 308 (6th Cir. 1985). *cert. denied,* 474 U.S. 1059 (1986).

Moore v. Provident Life and Accident Insurance Co., 786 F. 2d 922 (9th Cir. 1986).

National Association of Insurance Commissioners. (1989). *Model Health Maintenance Organization Act.* Washington, DC: Author.

National Center for Policy Analysis. (1988). *Freedom of choice in health insurance.* Dallas, TX. Author.

National Health Lawyers Association. (1989, November). Fewer HMOs leaving Medicare. *Health Lawyers News Report,* p. 6.

Northern Group Services v. Auto Owners Insurance Co., 833 F. 2d 85 (6th Cir. 1987).

Oregon Psychological Association v. Physicians Association of Clackamas County. Civil Action No. A8906-03626, Multnomah County Circuit Court (1989).

Oregon Revised Statutes. OR Rev. Stat. §§ 743.123, 743.556 (1975).

Sweede v. CIGNA Healthplan of Delaware, Inc., Civil Action No. 87C-SE-171-1CV (1988).

Tax Equity and Fiscal Responsibility Act of 1982, 42 U.S.C. § 1395 (1987).

Teti v. U.S. Healthcare, Inc., Civil Action #88-9808, United States District Court, Pennsylvania (1989).

Wells, K. B., Hays, R. D., Burnam, A., Rogers, W., Greenfield, S., & Ware, J. E. (1989, December). Detection of depressive disorder for patients receiving prepaid or fee-for-service care. *Journal of the American Medical Association,* 3298–3302.

Wickline v. State of California, 239 Cal. Rptr. 805, 741 P.2d 613 (1987).

Wilson v. Blue Cross of Southern California, 271 Cal. Rptr. 876 (Cal. App. 2 Dist. 1990).

5

Recent Managed-Care Legislative and Legal Issues

Shirley Ann Higuchi

The information in this chapter is an extension of Newman and Bricklin's review (chapter 4 in this book) of relevant legal issues concerning managed mental health care. These authors discussed the legislative, common-law, ethical, and professional practice guidelines regarding managed care. They noted that the managed-care legislation to date has established few parameters for ensuring the delivery of quality mental health services. As a result, enabling statutes, in the absence of stronger regulatory measures, have had an adverse impact on the delivery of health care. Newman and Bricklin also suggested cost-containment strategies that may be less compromising to quality mental health care.

First I describe the kinds of provisions that are typically contained in state statutes regarding utilization review, preferred provider organizations, and health maintenance organizations. Wherever possible, I point up those provisions that mental health professionals should be especially aware of. This information is based on my ongoing research for the Legal and Regulatory Affairs (LRA) office of the American Psychological Association's (APA) Practice Directorate, which entails evaluating state laws to discern whether and what provisions exist that may be applicable to the psychology profession. Next I discuss recent court cases in the area of managed care and the concept of expanding liability for managed-care systems and providers. Following that discussion, I describe some typical legal dilemmas faced by psychologists, most notably, those involving utilization review and access to mental health care services, and I illustrate these dilemmas with descriptions of actual complaints. I also discuss two emerging legal issues (exclusion from PPO panels and no-cause termination) that may be particularly relevant to providers and offer some advice for pursuing claims in those two arenas. Finally, I suggest a number of legal strategies that can be used by practitioners who are experiencing problems in managed-care systems, and I discuss the advantages and disadvantages of joining a managed-care entity.

I thank Rodney L. Lowman for his extensive editorial assistance and Robert J. Resnick for his helpful comments. I also thank legal interns Jodi Nadler, Neela Agarwalla, Todd M. Krim, and Eric Harris, who provided valuable legal research and input for this chapter.

Utilization Review Legislation

Utilization review (UR) involves the evaluation of the necessity, appropriateness, and efficiency of the use of health care services and resources. According to proponents of UR (e.g., managed-care entities and UR companies), its purpose is to improve cost-effectiveness while maintaining high quality of care and reducing abuse of services. As the UR industry rapidly expands, thereby affecting more practitioners and more patients, it becomes essential that uniform standards be established to ensure quality of care. Although many states have begun to adopt legislation in an effort to regulate the UR industry, no model statute currently exists. A "model statute" is typically a standard or sample statute proposed by a professional association or similar entity. Frequently, the state adopting the model act will modify it to some extent to meet its own needs or may adopt only a portion of the act (Black, 1979). However, several national associations, such as the newly established Utilization Review Accreditation Commission, a voluntary accrediting body, have circulated draft model provisions for inpatient UR. My staff and I reviewed existing state UR laws and found that several states' statutes (e.g., Georgia, Texas, and Hawaii) do contain provisions that are generally favorable to mental health practice. Most such laws, however, lack provisions that fully address the concerns of practitioners and fully protect the consumer.

Standard Provisions

Almost all of the UR legislation that my staff and I evaluated contains standard provisions that are intended to promote the delivery of quality health care in a cost-effective manner. As a result, the "purposes" sections of these statutes typically advocate greater coordination among health care providers, third-party payors, and UR or managed-care entities. Furthermore, the statutes seek to protect patients in several ways: (a) by ensuring that UR agents have the proper qualifications to perform UR, (b) by promoting public access to criteria and standards used in UR, and (c) by attempting to ensure the confidentiality of patients' medical records.

In addition, all statutes generally provide that an application and fee be submitted to the state regulating agency, which is typically identified as the state department of insurance, in order for the UR company to register for state certification. Generally, rules and regulations are promulgated by the state's insurance commissioner. Statutes provide that the commissioner has the authority to establish reporting requirements to evaluate the effectiveness of a UR entity's activities and to determine whether the entity is complying with the statutory requirements. As a result, the department of insurance may refuse to issue or renew a license, and it may suspend or revoke the payor's license or registration for noncompliance with the statutory provisions or regulations.

The standard provisions in UR laws require that the UR entity provide the patient or insured with a copy of the UR plan, including specific review criteria, standards, procedures, and methods to be used in the evaluation of proposed services. Many statutes also require that the UR entity establish a comprehensive appeals procedure by which the insured or the provider may seek review of an adverse decision. Moreover, UR entities must provide for the confidentiality of the patient or insured's medical records and personal information in accordance with applicable state and federal laws. Most statutes additionally require free telephone access for the patient or insured during regular business hours and additional arrangements for nonbusiness hours and for emergency situations. The statutes also typically require that the state insurance commissioner develop a formal complaint mechanism by which a provider may request that the commissioner conduct an investigation of the UR entity's review procedures in a particular case. It is important for psychologists to review carefully their individual state laws to determine whether they contain specific standards that may be used as an advocacy tool for the psychologist and the consumer. A key provision that may be helpful for psychologists to review in their state laws is the definition of what constitutes a "health care provider" for purposes of performing initial URs or reviews on appeal. Psychologists may obtain copies of statutes and regulations from their state insurance department.

The Like-Provider Provision

In some statutes, the definition of *health care provider* is ambiguous in terms of who is professionally qualified to conduct UR, whereas some statutes specifically mandate that the reviewer be a medical physician. It is important for mental health professionals to examine their state's UR legislation to determine whether their disciplinary groups are specifically excluded from qualification to perform UR. Some UR laws require that mental health UR be performed by an experienced mental health professional, rather than an insurance analyst or medical generalist. This requirement is specified by a like-provider provision, and it applies to initial reviews as well as appeal procedures. States must develop standards that provide for the delivery of quality health care and protect patients by ensuring that the reviewer is qualified to perform the UR and is similarly licensed with the same scope of practice as the provider. Such reviewers must have expertise in the identified review area as well. If a state specifically includes a like-provider provision (i.e., only those health care providers who are trained and licensed in the specific area in which the review is being conducted may make final determinations regarding services rendered or to be rendered), then psychologists have grounds for pressing UR or insurance companies to have psychologists on their review panels.

Other provisions that might be helpful to mental health professionals include those that establish parameters for conducting telephone reviews. Some states' UR laws have provisions regarding how reviewers may contact the attending providers and how reviewers identify themselves. The states' department of insurance may promulgate regulations requiring that the UR entity comply with applicable state and federal laws protecting patient confidentiality. Attending providers should also determine whether there are any provisions that ensure a provider's access to the UR reports before the reports are finalized.

Consumer Protection Provisions

Mental health professionals should also be aware of whether their state's UR laws include confidentiality provisions. Such requirements can be used to require UR entities to comply with whatever confidentiality terms the laws impose. These may include patient authorization for the release of records or limits on the amount of information that may be made available to third-party payors. Inquiry should also be made as to whether there are any statutory prohibitions regarding disclosure or publication of individual medical records or any other confidential information obtained in the performance of UR. The following is an example of a statutory provision derived from the *Illinois Revised Statutes* (1986) ensuring confidentiality of patient records:

> Any UR entity must include a program of utilization review which provides that all reviews be conducted by only those health care providers trained and licensed in the specific area in which the review is being conducted.

A statute might also contain a provision specifying that a reviewing professional or agent may not have any financial incentive that is in any way connected with the reviewer's decision to approve the health care services (e.g., length of stay, treatment chosen, or treatment setting). The UR entity may be required by law to provide the department of insurance with certification that there is no financial incentive, direct or indirect, that might influence the UR determination by the private reviewing agent.

Review decisions must be based on criteria that take into account necessary medical or psychological circumstances. Standards should also limit the frequency of specific case review to a level that does not interfere with the patient's care because a patient's uncertainty about when his or her next session will be authorized could prove countertherapeutic. Attending providers should be aware of statutory UR criteria and the UR processes being used. Statutes should be assessed to determine whether the review criteria are available to the treating provider.

Other important provisions are those that establish mechanisms for both providers and consumers to file complaints and those that regulate reporting of complaints to the insurance commissioner. Reporting requirements ensure that the department of insurance receives results of the reviews as well as the numbers and results of any appeals or complaints that have been filed. Therefore, if psychologists or patients contact the department of insurance with a complaint, then the commissioner, informed of any prior similar complaints, may be able to take appropriate actions.

Preferred Provider Organization Legislation

With increasing national concern over spiraling health care costs, the development of preferred provider organizations (PPOs) as an alternative to the traditional fee-for-service model of health care delivery has been rapidly expanding. As a result, states have begun not only to recognize such managed-care entities but also to increase the regulatory activity of these entities through uniform standards and requirements set forth in state legislation. PPOs (sometimes also called preferred provider arrangements or PPAs) are health care financing and delivery programs that provide financial incentives to consumers to use a preselected group of providers of health care. Payment to providers is typically on a fee-for-service basis, with discounts offered by the provider in exchange for guarantees of increased patient volume and quick reimbursement (Boochever, 1986). Consumers are usually not locked into receiving services from those preferred providers but have financial incentives to do so. Higher levels of coinsurance or deductibles routinely apply to services provided by nonparticipating providers.

PPOs pose significant challenges to practicing mental health professionals and consumers. Certain practices and policies of PPOs may restrict the delivery of mental health care only to selected classes of providers or may refer patients in need of mental health services only to physicians. Because subscribers receive most initial treatment from a primary care physician, some providers can be denied the opportunity to become fully participating members in that physicians may not choose to refer patients to certain types of providers. Furthermore, PPOs may be exempt from state laws that prohibit discrimination against certain classes of providers and certain consumer groups (e.g., state-mandated benefits and freedom-of-choice laws). In addition, available levels of mental health coverage provided in various PPO plans are minimal and fail to meet the needs of certain patients. As a result, patients may be forced to forego necessary treatment, pay for services out of pocket, or obtain services from the public sector.

Although many states' PPO statutes and regulations contain provisions that are generally favorable to the practice of psychology (discussed later in this section), other state laws (e.g., Annotated Statutes of Minnesota, 1986; Kentucky Administrative Regulations, 1991; Nebraska Revised Statutes, 1987) do not adequately address the concerns of either psychologists or consumers. Furthermore, because the PPO is a relatively new type of managed care, many states have yet to formally recognize or regulate such an arrangement. Of those states that have provided for PPOs in their health care or insurance laws, only a few have provided for more than a basic enabling statute or minimal regulatory guidelines (e.g., Annotated Laws of Massachusetts, 1981; Arkansas Code Annotated, 1987). In those states in which no specific PPO law exists, the PPO enabling and regulatory language may be found within other health service statutes. Those who are reviewing statutes should be aware that a thorough search of the state code may be necessary to determine regulatory control mechanisms for PPOs.

Standard Provisions

Most of the PPO or PPA legislation that my staff and I reviewed contain standard provisions that enable providers to enter contractual agreements with a group, and sometimes individual purchasers, to provide for alternative rates of payment specified in advance for a defined period of time. PPAs are generally the same as PPOs; however, a PPO tends to identify the entity itself, whereas the term *PPA* usually refers to the contractual or structural arrangement of the PPO. According to the statutes, the purpose of these enactments is to assist in the overall effort to reduce the cost of providing health care services. Traditionally, there exists a system by which payment terms are negotiated according to a fee-for-service model that often allows a discount. The negotiated payment rates are almost always accompanied by a waiver of coinsurance and deductibles for patients. Many statutes require that the PPO initially register with the state's department of insurance. Once registered, the PPO must provide for the continuous quality of care; the performance of medical personnel; and the utilization of services, facilities, and costs. The PPO must establish administrative procedures for management information systems, claims processing, and quality assurance.

The more comprehensive PPO statutes provide for state insurance commissioners to promulgate regulations designed to ensure accessibility of provider services to individuals within an insured group. These regulations are intended to ensure that the number and locations of institutional facilities and professional providers are adequate and that providers are appropriately licensed. Furthermore, state statutes often insist that PPO policies and contracts be consistent with standards of good health care and that all contracts with providers and facilities be fair and reasonable.

Some PPO laws have standard provisions requiring that the PPO cover and reimburse patients for the services of nonpreferred providers. Under this arrangement, nonpreferred providers do not have a formal contracting arrangement with the PPO, and they are considered nonpanel providers. The incentive for the patient to see a panel provider is typically financial, in the form of discounted fees, minimal copayments, and perhaps the absence of a deductible. In contrast, reimbursement for the services of a nonpanel provider is typically an indemnity arrangement whereby the patient is responsible for a deductible and a copayment. The PPO may, for example, cover 80% of the provider's usual and customary fee, whereas the patient is responsible for a 20% copayment. Furthermore, most PPO laws have a provision that payment for emergency care is not dependent on whether services are performed by a preferred or a nonpreferred provider.

Antidiscrimination Provisions

Many statutes include provisions that govern the terms and conditions that PPOs set for providers who seek to enter into a preferred provider arrangement. Freedom-of-choice, willing-provider, and antidiscrimination provisions are intended to protect both providers and consumers from discrimination and to ensure variety and quality of service delivery. Willing-provider and antidiscrimination provisions typically state that qualified providers who are willing to accept a PPO's terms and conditions cannot be excluded as a class from that PPO's panel. Freedom-of-choice provisions typically prohibit exclusive provider arrangements. These types of provisions are also intended to ensure that provider panels consist of a variety of providers with appropriate expertise and that patients have access to the type of health care services suited to their individual needs.

However, in some PPO statutes these provisions are modified such that premiums, conditions, and benefits for particular types of services may differ. Advocates for both psychologists and the consumer population need to be cognizant of these issues when reviewing proposed or actual PPO legislation. Thus, psychologists should review carefully the insurance-related legislation in their states to determine, first, whether PPO laws exist, and, second, whether specific revisions need to be made that can assist psychologists in obtaining better benefits for the consumer. As with UR legislation, it is important to look at the statutory definitions section to see whether a particular provider group is defined as a health care provider for the purposes of providing services. If a PPO is not required, for example, to have psychologists as panel members, then psychologists may be at a disadvantage. Therefore, it is necessary to be aware of any exclusive provider arrangements or prohibitions, in addition to any excessive copayment or deductible provisions, if the PPO plan must provide for reimbursement to nonpreferred providers.

Consumer Protection Provisions

PPOs must fully inform consumers regarding covered services, including any limitations and exclusions. Consumers should also be provided with a clear description of the formal grievance procedures in the event that they have a complaint. Ideally, PPOs should also have marketing and education programs that clearly and fully disclose information regarding referral services, utilization and quality-control mechanisms, and financial incentives used by providers to contain costs. For example, consumers should be informed of the existence of incentive plans whereby a provider's decision to refer a patient to a specialist may be based on how much income that provider will receive from the plan. Consumers need this kind of information to be able to make educated decisions about the attending provider's referral recommendations. Common in PPO legislation are truth-in-advertising provisions and provisions requiring full disclosure of information to consumers, particularly in regard to financial arrangement and cost-control mechanisms.

Providers should review their state's PPO legislation to determine whether a provision exists prohibiting excessive financial incentives for consumers who use the services of preferred provider participants. These provisions may appropriately require that no provider be permitted to hold any financial incentive that is bound to a decision to approve of health care services as a cost-containment measure.

The maximum level of mental health services currently prescribed in PPO plans may be inadequate in many situations. Easily accessible and appropriate mental health services provided by licensed psychologists and other mental health professionals can help prevent overuse of more costly medical services and ensure that consumers are receiving adequate mental health care by fully trained experts (Dickstein, Hanig, & Grosskopf, 1988). The problem of inadequate provision of mental health care may be addressed by requiring PPOs to submit to the department of insurance a report on the PPO's UR program that shows compliance with the general requirements set forth in the state UR law. It is important for mental health professionals to be informed of any requirements that affect the PPO's UR procedures. Moreover, statutory provisions may require that mental health services offered through PPOs be provided by licensed professionals and require that specific disciplinary groups be represented on UR panels. The following quote from the Illinois Revised Statutes (1986) is an example of such a provision:

> Any PPO providing hospital, medical, dental, or other health care services must include a program of utilization review which provides that all reviews be conducted by only those health care providers trained and licensed in the specific area in which the review is being conducted.

It is desirable that PPO statutes include strict confidentiality requirements. State statutes should be reviewed to determine whether provisions exist requiring the patient's authorization to release treatment records. Preferred confidentiality provisions are similar to those discussed regarding UR statutes. In addition, provisions for strict penalties for any breach of confidentiality are desirable, such as the following:

> The PPO shall ensure that the confidential relationship between the provider and the patient is safeguarded pursuant to state and federal law. Information pertaining to the diagnosis, treatment, or health of any person receiving health care benefits shall be confidential and shall not be disclosed to any person, except to the extent that it may be necessary to carry out the purposes of this Act. All information released to the PPO administrator shall require prior patient authorization. (Michigan Compiled Laws Annotated, 1988, p. 12)

The confidentiality privilege rests with the patient. Therefore, if a patient consents to release information to the PPO for claims processing, then the provider must make that information available. Often a psychologist may believe that the information requested by a managed-care entity is overinclusive and goes beyond the bounds of what is considered necessary. If that is the case, then the psychologist should explain the nature of the request to the client and indicate whether the psychologist believes that the request is within the bounds of acceptability, before the information is released.

PPO statutes should also be examined to determine whether a provision exists requiring PPOs to report annually to the insurance commissioner. The report should include information regarding the number of persons receiving benefits, the number of preferred providers, and the volume of business conducted during the year. With such statutory reporting requirements, psychologists may be able to obtain specific information to use in influencing the PPO's provision of mental health services.

Health Maintenance Organization Legislation

The health maintenance organization (HMO) is perhaps the most well known of the managed-care models. For a predetermined, capitated premium, the HMO delivers, or arranges for the delivery of, carefully managed and controlled health care services to a set number of individual clients (Boochever, 1986). This unique combination in which the insurer or the arranger of health care is also the provider of health care services raises some inherent conflicts that can be problematic for professionals contracting to provide services in such managed-care organizations.

Because the licensure and regulation of an HMO takes place at the state level, providers need to be aware of the HMO laws in their particular state. Furthermore, although the federal Health Maintenance Organization Act of 1973 and federal regulators continue to police Medicare and Medicaid operations, states have increasingly assumed responsibility for assessing the breadth of benefit selection, provider access, quality of care delivered to enrollees, and fiscal liability of prepaid health plans (Boochever, 1986). HMOs are required to be licensed or certified at the state level. Participation in federal programs under the Health Maintenance Organization Act of 1973 and the Tax Equity and Fiscal Responsibility Act of 1982 is voluntary.

Standard Provisions

The National Association of Insurance Commissioners (NAIC) has promulgated a Model Health Maintenance Organization Act for state licensure (NAIC, 1989). Approximately one fourth of the states have adopted the model in whole or in part. My staff and I found that virtually all HMO laws contain certain standard provisions. Although some of these provisions do not appear to be favorable to either psychologists or consumers, additional provisions could be incorporated into most HMO laws in order to protect these two groups.

The department of insurance or department of health in each state is frequently empowered to promulgate regulations to enforce HMO statutes and to permit the regulators to enforce these provisions. Almost all of the HMO laws include a definitions section that sets forth the general contents of the legislation. In addition, the state statutes outline the function of the department of insurance and provide information concerning evidence of coverage and a group health maintenance contract. HMOs are generally defined specifically so that those entities that are acting or operating like an HMO are required to be licensed at the state level. Furthermore, a standard HMO provision outlines the procedure that an HMO applicant must follow in order to be licensed at the state level, as well as the procedure to seek approval from the insurance commissioner.

For the most part, HMOs are required to submit basic organizational documents, including articles of incorporation or partnership agreements, contracts made by, or to be made by, any provider of health services, and statements generally describing the HMO's facilities and personnel. State laws usually require that any group contract, individual contract, evidence of coverage, or marketing materials be forwarded to the department of insurance. Such standard provisions allow the department of insurance or health to help ensure that these contracts are not onerous or unfair to the consumer population. The statutes also typically require financial statements to determine an HMO's assets, liabilities, and sources of financial support. These provisions are extremely important in the event that the department of insurance or health determines that the HMO is not fiscally viable to operate in that state as an HMO and thus cannot guarantee health care services to its enrollees. Another standard provision that serves to protect the consumer is a "protection against insolvency" provision. This requires HMOs to guarantee that the obligations to the enrollees of the HMO can be performed.

HMO statutes use "basic health care services" to define the various services that an HMO is required to cover. These services generally include inpatient hospital, physician, outpatient medical, laboratory, radiological, and preventive health services. The HMO Act requires HMOs to offer at least 20 outpatient mental health visits per year under basic benefits. It is very important to ensure that mental health, mental illness, and substance abuse treatment are also incorporated into the state law's definition of basic health services (as opposed to supplemental services). For example, some states (e.g., District of Columbia Code Annotated, 1993; Georgia Code Annotated, 1990; Revised Statutes Annotated of Arizona, 1992) provide mandatory mental health coverage, whereas other states (e.g., Annotated Code of Maryland—Health, 1991; Arkansas Code Annotated, 1987; Michigan Compiled Laws Annotated, 1988) do not. All of the statutes reviewed require HMOs to establish and maintain a reasonable procedural system by which written complaints may be resolved. In most states, these systems must be approved by the department of insurance. Most HMO statutes contain a section that prohibits HMOs from performing certain types of activities. Most HMO statutes prohibit advertising that is untrue or misleading or soliciting any form of marketing material that becomes misleading or deceptive. Most statutes use the "reasonable person" standard whereby information is judged to be misleading if a person who has no special knowledge of the health care coverage would construe the information as misleading or false. The significance of the information to the enrollee or potential enrollee is also used as an evaluation standard.

Most "prohibited practices" provisions also state that an HMO may not cancel or refuse to renew an enrollee's coverage on the basis of the enrollee's health status once he or she is enrolled. HMOs are also generally prohibited from discrimination against race, creed, color, sex, or religion in the selection or participation of health care providers in the HMO. Moreover, in some statutes, there are provisions prohibiting HMOs from discriminating against physicians as a class or against any class of providers that are enumerated. Such provisions are especially important for psychologists and other nonmedical providers.

State laws require HMOs to provide a definition of "basic health care services." By law, the HMO must provide any service that is included in its definition. An HMO may or may not include mental health or drug and alcohol abuse services in its definition of basic health care services. "Health care provider" and "health care professional" are defined in several different ways in HMO laws. For example, the Maryland Health–General Code (Annotated Code of Maryland—Health, 1991) defines "provider" to mean "any person, including the physician or hospital, who is licensed or otherwise authorized in the state to provide health care services."

Antidiscrimination Provisions

Similar to PPO legislation, most HMO statutes contain some type of freedom-of-choice or antidiscrimination provision. Antidiscrimination provisions typically prohibit HMOs from discriminating on the basis of race, creed, color, sex, or religion in the selection of health care providers for participation. However, some antidiscrimination provisions further stipulate that HMOs shall not unreasonably discriminate against physicians as a class or against any class of health care providers when contracting for specialty or referral practitioners.

Some HMO laws also include willing-provider or freedom-of-choice provisions. For example, many of the HMO statutes indicate through a willing-provider provision that the HMO shall not discriminate solely on the basis of the class to which the health professional belongs. In the event that the provider desires to join the HMO, and he or she is licensed in a particular area, the HMO cannot deny access based on his or her professional identification. With respect to freedom-of-choice provisions, some statutes indicate that an HMO must make the services available for specific mandated mental health professions (e.g., psychiatrists, psychologists, licensed independent clinical social workers, and clinical specialists in psychiatric and mental health nursing).

Consumer Protection Provisions

HMOs may offer a capitated arrangement whereby health care services are delivered on the basis of predetermined costs approved in advance by the insurance commissioner. However, state laws may stipulate that no financial incentive shall be so excessive as to essentially negate coverage and that HMOs not establish an exclusive provider arrangement such that consumers are all but forced into choosing a particular provider or group of providers. Furthermore, individual statutes should be reviewed to determine whether a provider is permitted to hold a financial incentive that is tied to any UR determinations.

After reviewing marketing materials and benefits booklets, my staff and I have concluded that information regarding financial arrangements and cost-containment mechanisms is not always fully disclosed to consumers. For example, it is clear that HMOs fail to inform consumers of their use of any physicians' incentive plans that link a provider's decision to refer the consumer to a particular specialist to how much income that physician will receive from the plan. HMOs may also be required by statute to provide educational materials to consumers fully disclosing information regarding the referral services, utilization and quality-control mechanisms, and financial incentives used in cost-control efforts. In addition to this information, consumers may request a copy of the formal grievance procedures to be used in the event that the consumer has a complaint with the HMO's activities. Mental health professionals should, therefore, review their state HMO law to determine whether it has specific disclosure requirements.

As with PPOs, the problem regarding the inadequate provision of mental health care may be addressed by requiring HMOs to submit to the state's department of insurance a UR plan that complies with the general requirements of the state's UR law. In addition, statutory provisions may or may not require that mental health services be provided by licensed professionals and that psychologists be represented on UR panels.

As with PPOs and UR entities, it is desirable that HMOs ensure the confidentiality of patients' records. Strict confidentiality provisions requiring the patient's authorization prior to the release of any treatment records must be enforced. Ideally, the same confidentiality requirements provided for in the state's UR statute should be made applicable to the HMO. In addition, statutes often include strict penalties for any violations of confidentiality.

As in the UR and PPO statutes, HMO laws may contain a reporting requirements provision to foster regulation of the HMOs by the state's insurance commissioners. The annual report to the commissioner typically includes information regarding the number of subscribers, the number and types of licensed providers, the volume of business conducted during the calendar year, and a financial statement that demonstrates the fiscal viability of the HMO.

Recent Court Cases Pertaining to Managed Care

In a managed-care system, providers are not always able to provide or obtain care that they believe is necessary for their patients, even when that care would appear to be covered by their patients' insurance (Appelbaum, 1993). If a UR entity concludes that the recommended care suggested by a mental health professional is not "medically necessary" (the standard ordinarily applied), then coverage may be denied, even if the patient has not exhausted available benefits (Brodman, 1993). It is clear that the failure of UR or managed-care companies to authorize coverage for providers' patients could create problems for those providers.

In chapter 4, Newman and Bricklin focused on certain parameters created by case law in the area of managed-care liability. They reviewed *Wickline v. State of California* (1987), which addressed physical and not mental health care liability in managed-care contexts. The case, which was upheld by the California Court of Appeals, identified the legal responsibility of a third-party payor for harm caused to a patient when a cost-containment mechanism is applied in a manner that affects the implementation of the provider's clinical judgment about required or desirable care. In *Wickline*, the court stated that the physician who complies without protest with the limitations imposed by a third-party payor when the provider's medical judgment dictates otherwise cannot avoid ultimate responsibility for the patient's care. As a result, this case is frequently cited in support of the proposition that when an attending provider disagrees with the position taken by the reviewing entity, the provider has an obligation aggressively to appeal the UR determination. Moreover, the court stated that payors can be held liable for negative outcomes if the reimbursement policies are negligently designed. In *Wickline*, however, the physician was held to be at fault because he had not protested adamantly against the dismissal of his patient from the hospital. The *Wickline* decision created a foundation for the imposition of liability for negligent utilization management decisions.

This concept of liability was expressed further by the same California court in *Wilson v. Blue Cross of Southern California* (1990). In *Wilson*, a patient was admitted to a psychiatric hospital while suffering from major depression, drug dependency, and anorexia. His treating physician determined that he needed 3–4 weeks of inpatient care. After 11 days of inpatient care, the UR company advised the insurer that it should not pay for more inpatient care. The patient was discharged, and 20 days later he committed suicide. The family sued both the insurer and the UR company. The UR company, Western Medical, specifically asserted that it was not liable under *Wickline* (1987) and sought to put the entire responsibility on the attending physician. The court rejected that effort because the case was brought against the insurer, not the physician. At a minimum, the alleged failure of the attending physician to follow Western Medical's informal policy requesting reconsideration was found not to warrant granting summary judgment. Summary judgment in this instance occurs when a party to a civil action is permitted to move for summary judgment on a claim when he or she believes that there is no genuine issue of material fact and that he or she is entitled to prevail as a matter of law (Black, 1979). The *Wilson* court specifically disagreed with *Wickline* on causation, observing that, in a multiple causation case, tort liability exists when the defendant's actions are a "substantial factor" in the injury. By way of background, a tort constitutes a private or civil wrong or injury, other than breach of contract, for which the court will provide a remedy in the form of action for damages (Black, 1979). The court also observed that, in most utilization management program cases, it is difficult to argue that a decision to deny coverage is not a substantial factor in the decision to discharge. The *Wilson* decision suggests that, in the future, UR entities could have difficulty obtaining summary judgments in negligence actions on the grounds that the denial of coverage is not a sufficient cause of the alleged injury to the beneficiary. Undoubtedly, there will be litigation seeking to balance the duties for UR entities suggested by *Wilson* and *Wickline* with the implied right of an insurer to review medical-necessity determinations that are made by the treating physician.

A recent case from the U.S. Court of Appeals further reaffirmed the holdings in *Wickline* and *Wilson*. In *Corcoran v. United Health Care* (1992), a woman was in a category of high-risk pregnancy. Her doctor ordered hospitalization with complete bed rest. United Health Care determined that hospitalization was unnecessary but authorized 10 hours per day of home nursing care. The baby died while the nurse was off duty, and the mother sued United Health Care for negligence. The court cited *Wilson* and *Wickline* for their new and limited recognition of a cause for action against third-party payors. The court ultimately decided that the issue was preempted by the Employee Retirement Income Security Act (ERISA) of 1974, but it did recognize that United Health Care made "medical decisions as part and parcel of its mandate to decide what benefits are available" (cited in Steele, 1992, pp. 2–6). ERISA is a federal law that preempts state laws for self-insured employee benefit plans. However, it contains an "insurance savings clause" that excepts from preemption those state laws which "regulate insurance." This issue is becoming increasingly important as employee benefit plans try to evade the state-mandated benefit provisions or provider laws (i.e., willing provider and freedom-of-choice provisions) by claiming preemption under ERISA (see chapter 4 in this book).

In addition to liability stemming from utilization management and quality assurance issues, managed-care entities can be liable for "bad-faith" claim denials. Bad-faith claim denials can exist even when there is no allegation of negligence on the part of the treating physicians or hospitals (Harbaugh, 1993). In *Hughs v. Blue Cross of Northern California* (1989), a patient's claim for payment of hospitalization benefits for severe psychiatric problems was denied by his mother's employer's health plan. After further investigation, it was revealed that the discharge summary and attending physician's history of treatment and diagnosis records were all missing from the claims file. The plaintiff (patient) successfully argued that there was no evidence that the missing records had ever been reviewed. The decision for compensatory and punitive damages totaling $850,000 was later upheld in appeals court (Harbaugh, 1993).

Relatedly, a Louisiana UR case was upheld by the U.S. Court of Appeals ruling that the defendant abused its discretion when terminating inpatient psychiatric care benefits for a patient (*Salley v. E. D. DuPont de Nemours & Company*, 1992). In *Salley*, the issue was not what the plan administrator knew of the patient's claim at the time he made the decision but what data that administrator failed to obtain. In order to make an informed decision regarding the *Salley* claim, the plan administrator should have sought additional records on her case.

Liability for managed-care entities is expanding under the theories of respondant superior, ostensible agency, corporate liability, and breach of contract. Staff-model HMOs most frequently are subject to the theory of respondant superior. This doctrine states that a higher authority is responsible for the actions taken on its behalf. When the providers are direct employees of an HMO, it is not difficult to find the HMO liable for employees' misdeeds. This was apparent in the case of *Sloan v. Metropolitan Health Council of Indianapolis, Inc.* (1987), in which a medical malpractice action was brought against an HMO, alleging negligent failure to diagnose. The court held that there was a material issue of disputed fact as to whether the usual requisites of an agency or employer–employee relationship existed, and the court thereby precluded summary judgment on the issue of whether the HMO was vicariously liable for malpractice by the employee-physician. The court further held that the HMO cannot avoid liability under the doctrine of respondeat superior simply by failing to incorporate under the state's professional corporation act. In other words, although the entity did not register as a corporation under the relevant state laws, the entity would still be viewed as a professional corporation for purposes of liability. There was evidence that Metropolitan's staff physicians were under the control of its medical director, a physician, who policed medical services and established policy. The circumstances of the case established that an employment relationship existed where the employee performed acts within the scope of his employment. The practice of medicine by Metropolitan was found to be equivalent to the practice of medicine by a professional corporation. In sum, the court ruled that where the usual requisites of agents to an employer–employee relationship exist, a corporation may be held vicariously liable for malpractice for the acts of its employee-physicians.

Schleier v. Kaiser Foundation Health Plan (1989) was another case in which respondeat superior was applied. In this case, the defendant was held liable for the actions of a physician who was not under any type of contract but was simply a consulting specialist. The key element in assigning liability was that the specialist had never directly informed the plaintiff that he was not affiliated with the HMO. The case was more or less a question of the legal principle of ostensible agency because it assigned liability based on a relationship that the plaintiff thought had existed but which, in fact, had not. Under the doctrine of ostensible agency, the issue is not whether or not an individual is actually contractually affiliated with a business entity but whether a reasonable consumer believes that the individual is affiliated with the business and relies on this belief. In *Schleier*, the personal representative of the deceased patient's estate brought an action under the District of Columbia's survival statute claiming that the HMO physicians treating the patient had negligently failed to diagnose and treat the patient's latent coronary disease. The court held that the HMO was vicariously liable for the negligence of its consulting physician, notwithstanding the HMO's argument that the physician was an independent contractor. Vicarious liability constitutes indirect legal responsibility, for example, liability of an employer for the acts of an employee (Black, 1979). The physician was brought in as a consultant by the HMO physician, and the HMO had some ability to control his behavior because the physician was responsible to the HMO physician. It further appeared that the physician's actions in providing the health care services in question fell within the HMO's "regular business."

Boyd v. Albert Einstein Medical Center (1988) is a case that directly applied the theory of ostensible agency to an HMO. The court did not impose liability based on respondeat superior. The defendant HMO did not employ the physician in question, who was being sued along with the HMO and hospital for an allegedly negligent breast biopsy that led to the death of a patient. The plan had specifically advertised that the physicians who worked with it were competent and carefully regulated. The court said that such advertising could lead the plaintiff to believe that the physician was an agent of the HMO. The court held that the HMO was liable under the ostensible agency theory because the treating physician was an agent of the HMO, and because the patient looked to the institution, rather than to the individual physician, for care. Furthermore, the HMO "held out" the physician as its employee. In the court's opinion, because the decedent was required to follow mandates of the HMO and had not directly sought the attention of a specialist, there was an inference that the plaintiff looked to the institution for care, and not solely to the physician. In addition, the decedent had submitted herself to the care of the participating physician in response to an invitation from the HMO; hence the HMO was liable for the acts of the physician. In *McClellan v. Health Maintenance Organization of Pennsylvania* (1992), the court ruled in favor of the plaintiff under the ostensible agency doctrine, because the HMO advertised that it carefully screened its primary care physicians.

Corporate negligence or corporate liability is another expanding area of managed-care liability. Corporate liability is ruled when courts disregard the usual immunity of corporate officers or entities from liability for corporate activities. As provider selection becomes a significant issue for managed-care entities, the theory of corporate liability will be applied to HMOs and PPOs in the future. A duty to protect the patient will arise when provider selection results in limiting and restricting a patient's choice of provider (Hinden & Elden, 1990). Hence, the HMO or PPO will have the duty to properly review and investigate the credentials and expertise of provider panel applicants. This view was expressed in *Harrell v. Total Health Care, Inc.* (1989), in which an HMO was held to have a nondelegable duty to enrollees to select physicians carefully. Furthermore, the HMO could be liable where, although it checked certain records, it did not personally interview the physicians or check their references.

Under the breach-of-contract theory, managed-care entities could be held liable for not living up to what they promised in their enrollee contracts or marketing materials. As was discussed earlier, in *Boyd v. Albert Einstein Medical Center* (1988), the court ruled that an HMO might be liable for the acts of contracting physicians in part because the HMO had advertised that its providers were competent and had been evaluated by the HMO. Furthermore, the HMO guaranteed the quality of the care provided to its enrollees. Therefore, marketing materials, enrollment contracts, and literature provided to the patient advertising certain guarantees are considered contractual agreements between managed-care entities and enrollees.

A managed-care entity may also be liable for breach of contract in other circumstances. Typically, a contract exists between the patient and a third-party payor to pay for medically necessary services (Becker, Tiano, & Marshall, 1992). Hence, an improper review decision that results in nonpayment is a direct breach of contract. Because denying authorization of treatment may result in the patient's foregoing medical services, the third-party payor may, depending on the circumstances, be liable for injury or death caused to the patient.

Typical Legal Dilemmas Faced by Managed Mental Health Care Providers

Over the past several years, the LRA office of APA's Practice Directorate has received frequent complaints by both providers and patients.

Questions have been raised regarding the quality of care delivered to patients, whether managed-care systems restrict access to care, and whether the cost-containment measures inherent in such systems are effective. Although LRA receives most of its inquiries from individual providers and state psychological associations, the office also receives calls directly from patients who are experiencing difficulties with managed-care organizations. Outside organizations have also sought information regarding psychology's involvement in managed-care settings. For example, employer groups, insurance companies, HMOs, and PPOs have contacted LRA regarding the practice of psychology as these groups seek standards or criteria to assist them in delivering psychological services. Similarly, this office receives informational inquiries from state and federal reimbursement programs. All data and information presented in this section have been gathered from the complaints and inquiries that have been directed to LRA during the past several years.

Although the types of complaints received by LRA vary from case to case, the issues typically can be classified into two categories: UR and accessibility to mental health care. As has been stated, all managed-care entities and insurance companies have UR programs. One common complaint is that managed-care entities employ poorly trained, sometimes unlicensed, personnel who are unfamiliar with the field of service in which they are empowered to review, perhaps because their primary focus is on cost containment rather than quality mental health services. As was discussed earlier, UR-related complaints have indeed recently surfaced in court. Managed-care entities can be liable for patients' injuries resulting from the entity's own negligence, and courts may find UR programs liable for recommending lengths of stay or discharge dates that harm the patient. Indeed, a third-party payor could be held liable for injuries resulting from an arbitrary or unreasonable decision to deny requests for medical care, particularly if it is not appealed (see *Wickline*, 1987; *Wilson*, 1990).

One of the most frequent and serious complaints raised in the UR arena pertains to what providers regard as unreasonable requests for information by UR companies. Ethical and practice dilemmas arise when raw data, progress notes, and other information beyond what is considered reasonable are requested from psychologists. Both providers and patients have complained about the lack of written or oral justification by UR entities when refusing to authorize additional coverage for services. As a result, mental health professionals are continuously searching for guidance regarding ethical and practice dilemmas when delivering services in a managed-care setting. Some states have begun to propose and implement legislation to help regulate UR activities.

Although it is true that some form of regulation may be desirable, some states' UR laws contain provisions that may adversely affect the practice of psychology. For example, the current Maryland law (Annotated Code of Maryland—Health, 1991) requires certification of private review agents who are performing UR activities on behalf of an insurance company. The certification requirements provide that a medical doctor must support and supervise the work of the reviewers. Maryland passed an amendment to this statute, however, specifically regarding UR of mental health care services. The amendment states that any determination to deny or reduce coverage of mental health care, and any final determination after an appeals process, must be made by a physician or by a panel containing a physician. The LRA office of APA's Practice Directorate contacted the Maryland Department of Insurance to obtain an interpretation of these provisions (personal communication, June 1990). The regulator indicated that the statute would not be likely to be literally interpreted as written, and that supervision of a licensed psychologist by a physician would not be required. Although this information is not conclusive, it may be indicative of how the Maryland state law will be applied. In any event, this type of legislation could adversely affect those programs in which qualified licensed psychologists review the services provided by other psychologists. Other states that have provisions requiring a physician's supervision or participation include Arkansas, Florida, Kentucky, Mississippi, South Carolina, and Virginia.

A second general area of complaint involves accessibility to psychological services. Typically, the practices and policies of managed-care entities restrict access in the delivery of mental health care and other services to consumers. This problem is compounded by the manner in which managed-care entities are designed and implemented. For example, difficulties are presented by the physician gatekeeping process when unrealistic limits are placed on mental health services through the use of caps on dollars spent and limits on number of visits allowed. Furthermore, the quality and appropriateness of mental health services provided through the managed-care entities are often considered by providers to be inadequate. Furthermore, consumers are often not provided full information about the operation of the managed-care plan and the financial arrangements offered by the managed-care entity. Specifically, managed-care plans often fail to fully disclose information about their cost-control mechanisms, such as the use of incentive plans that link a provider's decision to refer a patient to a specialist to how much income that provider will receive. Providers themselves may not be adequately informed about the managed-care system before entering into a legally binding relationship with a managed-care entity. Mental health care providers should be aware of potential accessibility problems and address any concerns to the provider-relations director of the organization prior to signing a contract with a managed-care entity.

Managed-care entities operating under ERISA have also been subject to complaint. It has been reported that some ERISA self-insured arrangements have directly excluded psychologists from being providers or, alternatively, have required a physician to supervise the work of the psychologist. (ERISA benefits are not bound by state mandates or freedom-of-choice laws.) Such practices further inhibit the patient's access to psychological services. In addition, these entities tend to limit the amount of covered services. In contrast, although experience indicates that HMOs and PPOs—which may or may not be affiliated with a self-insured arrangement—will include psychologists as participating providers, they may authorize only a limited number, thus limiting a consumer's access to his or her choice of provider and excluding newly licensed psychologists from participation.

Specific Examples of Typical Legal Dilemmas

Disruption of Care or Confidentiality

A frequent complaint brought to the attention of APA's Practice Directorate's LRA office concerns a situation in which one managed-care entity is merged with another health care corporation. Mergers, acquisitions, and corporate purchasing arrangements of existing plans can disrupt patient care and the continuity of care between providers and patients. For example, it came to the attention of LRA that a large corporation signed a contract with a managed mental health company to handle all of the corporation's mental health care services. This process has created some difficulties for those covered individuals who were already seeing a mental health care provider at the time the new plan took effect. The managed-care company gave mental health care providers the opportunity to participate as managed-care providers. However, problems could arise if the patient did not sign the contract, because the patient's insurance coverage would drop from 80% to only 50%. Obviously the ultimate choice for deciding to accept the terms of a managed-care entity rests with the provider. However, LRA suggested that the provider attempt to bring these concerns to the managed-care entity in an effort to seek a more equitable resolution.

Psychologists have also raised concerns that a managed-care company's system essentially relies on a medical model rather than a psychological one. In one situation, during the UR process, a managed-care company's reviewer recommended that a patient receive medication as part of his psychotherapy treatment. This recommendation, in the eyes of the therapist, could demonstrate interference in the provider–patient relationship.

Reviewing claims by telephone can also raise problems. In one instance, LRA was alerted to the fact that reviewers (who have had no direct contact with a patient) have suggested that a patient consult with a psychiatrist about the need for medication. If a patient refuses medication, then the reviewer may threaten a denial of insurance reimbursement on the basis that the patient has refused to follow "the best medical advice."

Managed-care entities are responsible for ensuring the confidentiality of patients' records. However, the experience of several practitioners has been that confidentiality provisions have been deficient. As one example, a practitioner informed LRA that he contacted the managed-care company by telephone through the provider-relations line, identifying himself as a psychologist who needed to ask a reviewer some questions regarding a patient whose case had been reviewed the previous week. The psychologist stated that he could not recall the reviewer's name, but could only remember her gender. The clerk proceeded to mention several names of female reviewers, none of which the psychologist recognized. In addition, the clerk asked for the patient's corporation employee number, and the psychologist indicated that he currently did not have this information with him. However, the provider was able to provide the name of the patient. The clerk pulled the patient's file onto the computer screen, confirmed that the employee was, in fact, in psychotherapy with the psychologist, provided the psychologist with the reviewer's name, and informed the psychologist that the reviewer was unavailable to speak with the psychologist at that time. The psychologist was disturbed by the ease with which any type of information concerning the patient could have been extracted from the clerk, or, potentially, the reviewer. The managed-care company had not established a system to verify that the person calling was, in fact, a bona fide provider treating the patient in question. In this case, as well as others, the provider can file a complaint with the managed-care entity, alerting it to the inadequacies of the review process.

By filing a complaint with a managed-care entity, the provider is able to alert the entity to the problem at hand, which, of course, gives the entity the opportunity to correct it. Most important, however, in the event that a legal challenge is instituted against the managed-care entity for its failure to abide by confidentiality rules, the provider should keep an accurate record of his or her dealings with the reviewer so as not to be seen as a participant in an ineffective system of maintaining patients' records.

A psychologist complained to LRA about a managed-care entity that handles and manages mental health benefits for employers and other groups. The psychologist was asked to sign a contract with the entity that stipulated that a representative of the entity be allowed to attend therapy sessions as long as the patient consented. This issue raises several practical and ethical dilemmas. The therapy session between the provider and the patient would probably be disrupted, because the patient is likely to be uncomfortable having an observer, particularly if that observer is not a qualified therapist. Moreover, regardless of whether the patient would willingly consent to this arrangement, a potential for financial coercion may exist. That is, if the client does not agree to allow the managed-care representative to observe the therapy session, the company may not reimburse the client for services rendered. In essence, the insurance company indirectly forces the patient to waive his or her confidentiality rights.

LRA did object to this provision and worked closely with state psychological associations to file complaints with both the state department of insurance and other governmental bodies. From a purely legal standpoint, the managed-care entity at issue may state that because it obtained client consent, illegal breaches of confidentiality did not exist. However, pressure was applied on the entity by citing bad business practices. In some instances, it appeared as if the managed-care entity removed the provisions in some of its provider contracts; however, LRA was recently informed that the entity still uses the contracts in some geographic locations.

Hold-Harmless Provisions

Many managed-care entities ask providers to sign contracts that contain "hold-harmless" provisions. Along with the other provisions in the contracts, these clauses are designed to differentiate the provider and the managed-care company as separate and independent entities, each of which is solely responsible for damages resulting from its own negligence. Essentially the provisions state that liability for a provider's services is covered under the provider's own malpractice policy. Under such a provision, the payor, managed-care entity, or any of their agents or representatives shall not be held liable for any cause of action or liability arising out of, or in connection with, services rendered by the provider.

An example of such a provision is as follows: Under the indemnification provision, a contract states that providers shall indemnify and hold the insurance company harmless from any and all claims, lawsuits, settlements, and liabilities incurred as a result of professional services provided or not provided by a provider with respect to any covered person. Relatedly, the insurance company shall indemnify and hold the provider harmless from any and all claims, lawsuits, settlements, and liabilities incurred as a result of actions taken or not taken by the insurance company in the administration of the employer's group health benefit plan. The intent in this provision appears to be that the provider agrees to indemnification for his or her negligence in providing or not providing services, and the company agrees to indemnification for negligence or other damages in connection with administration of the plan. Requiring the provider to assume responsibility for his or her own negligent conduct, to insure him- or herself against that responsibility, and to protect the managed-care company through indemnification for liability does not seem to be an unreasonable contractual arrangement. However, hold-harmless agreements need to be carefully reviewed to ensure that this appropriate intent is realized, especially in light of the *Wickline* case (1987), whereby both the managed-care company and the provider can be found negligent, either separately or jointly.

For example, one problematic clause that was brought to the attention of LRA was a provision in a contract that read as follows:

> Liability for Provider services are covered under Provider's own practice liability. The payor or [managed care entity] or any of their agents or representatives shall not be liable for any cause of action or liability arising out of or in connection with services rendered by the provider.

This contractual provision was, in the opinion of the LRA staff, poorly drafted and raised interpretative questions. The provision did not appear to create a true indemnity relationship, because it disclaimed liability rather than requiring the providing psychologist to indemnify against it. A court could construe the clause as an intended agreement to indemnify. However, another argument is that the agreement to indemnify was intended to cover damages that arise not only from the provider's own negligent conduct but also damages that arise from the managed-care company's negligent conduct, so long as that liability arises "in connection with services rendered by the provider."

In the foregoing examples, the hold-harmless provisions appear to be setting forth a subcontracting relationship between the managed-care entity and the provider. Such a relationship would limit each party's liabilities to its own respective actions. Other provisions have been brought to the attention of LRA that are even more ambiguous. For instance, one managed-care organization's plan contained a provision that stated that the specialist/provider will hold the managed care organization harmless due to any malpractice litigation and will have a minimum of one million dollars worth of professional liability insurance. Providers shall notify the managed care organization within 48 hours of loss of insurance.

If one were to read this provision literally, seemingly any malpractice claim that would arise could be included. In other words, the provider would be required to indemnify the managed-care organization even if the organization were partially at fault. Clearly these hold-harmless provisions would be unreasonable, because malpractice liability insurance typically covers only those specific acts arising out of the conduct of the provider. The provider cannot assume liability for other parties unless the provider directly arranges for such liability and agrees to take it on. The primary purpose of psychology malpractice liability insurance is to insure against damages resulting from the psychologist's negligence, not from the negligence of entities with which psychologists engage in business.

Verifying Contractual Definitions and Provisions

Many managed-care entities, through contractual arrangements, limit reimbursement to the therapist to only services that are deemed "medically necessary." These entities do not provide a definition of what constitutes a "medically necessary" service, and, as a result, the therapist is not given a sense, in advance, of what services are and are not covered.

An illustrative case that came to the attention of LRA concerns an insurance company whose actions may have unfairly denied necessary mental health services to a patient who was insured under the company's plan. It was alleged that the insurance company had reduced the patient's benefits based on its determination that the current treatment provided by the attending psychologist did not constitute a covered benefit under the plan. Although the psychologist appealed the insurance company's original decision, a second denial was issued after an evaluation. The purpose of this evaluation was to provide a second opinion in order to review more thoroughly the basis for the denial of benefits. A medical examination was arranged by the insurance company and performed by a certified psychiatrist chosen by the insurance company. After the medical evaluation, the insurance company determined that there was insufficient information to support the medical necessity of care at a frequency of three visits per week. Based on its predetermined criteria as it chose to interpret them here, the insurance company concluded that the benefits would continue for two visits per week and would be reduced to a 1-hr session per week within a couple of weeks. Subsequent to this reduction, the insurance company would perform a follow-up review.

One of the issues raised by this case was that the insurance company misquoted its own benefit package to the provider and the patient. The insurance company had stated in a letter to the provider that services that are recommended by a physician only, and are essential for the necessary care and treatment of any illness or injury, would be covered. However, this policy was not found in the benefit documents. It is important, therefore, that psychologists and their patients carefully review the written benefits plan and not rely solely on the payor's interpretation. In addition to advertising and marketing materials, benefit summary plans provided to the patient or insured constitute a contract between the patient or insured and the insurance company. It may need to be brought to the insurance company's attention by the psychologist that, essentially, any deviation from these contractual obligations could constitute a breach of contract between the patient or insured and the insurance company.

Conflict of Interest

Conflict-of-interest concerns have also commonly come to the attention of LRA. For example, when a psychologist is working for a corporation under an employee assistance plan (EAP), what happens if the psychologist owes a duty or responsibility both to the corporation who employs the psychologist and to the client? In one case, this issue arose when a psychologist, who was working in an EAP setting in a corporation, was informed by the employer that the provision of information or resources to employees on issues such as legal referrals, further mental health treatment, or tax assistance was appropriate. However, the corporation also informed the psychologist that in the event that the employee was contemplating legal action against the company, or if an issue such as sexual harassment arose, then the psychologist was not to provide resources to the patient regarding legal assistance. The *Ethical Principles of Psychologists and Code of Conduct* (APA, 1992a) specifically addresses this issue. Principle 8.03 states:

> If the demands of an organization with which psychologists are affiliated conflict with this Ethics Code, psychologists clarify the nature of the conflict, make known their commitment to the Ethics Code, and to the extent feasible, seek to resolve the conflict in a way that permits the fullest adherence to the Ethics Code. (p. 1610)

The *Ethical Principles* clearly indicate that in this situation the psychologist has an obligation to approach the corporation and seek clarification on what his or her obligations are to the corporation and to the client. Furthermore, it appears that the psychologist has a duty to inform the patient of any conflicts or compromising situations that can or will arise. Incidentally, as an employee of the organization, a psychologist would be in an excellent position to assist the company in developing standards in this area, as well as to clarify them for both the corporation and its employees.

Two Emerging Legal Issues for Psychologists in Managed-Care Settings

The Practice Directorate's LRA office receives several phone calls each month from psychologists concerned about two evolving legal issues that affect psychologists either presently involved in managed-care practice or considering participation in one. The first issue is the exclusion of psychologists from PPO panels. Generally speaking, there is not much that one can do individually to challenge a refusal of membership by a managed-care company, unless the exclusion is outright discriminatory. There are, however, certain steps that can be taken to determine whether these "closed provider panels" potentially violate a state law or regulation. The second issue is the "no-cause" termination provision found in many managed-care contracts. This provision stipulates that a managed-care company or the health care provider can terminate a provider's contract without having to justify the termination. In addition, the managed-care companies are not required to afford the provider an opportunity to appeal or challenge the termination. Following a discussion of each of these issues, I outline some recommended steps that psychologists can take in pursuing claims in these arenas.

Exclusion From Preferred Provider Organization Panels

As was previously stated, it is quite difficult to challenge a PPO's decision to refuse the application of a provider who wants to join the provider panel. In order to fully appreciate why such a claim would probably fail, one must understand some basic PPO concepts. Proponents of managed care would argue that a PPO provides health care in a more cost-effective manner than do indemnity plans. Providers are typically reimbursed on a discounted fee-for-service basis in exchange for a guarantee of increased patient volume and quick reimbursement payments. Although members are sometimes free to receive treatment from nonpreferred providers, higher copayments or deductibles serve as a financial disincentive to do so. A primary objective of the PPO is to provide financial incentives to its members to use the select group of preferred providers, thereby reducing costs. Thus PPO administrators contend that it would not make good business sense for a PPO to accept every psychologist who applies to the panel, when its objective is to foster competition among applicants for the best quality service at the lowest price. The cost savings are then passed on to the PPO members who utilize the preferred providers. In essence, this arrangement is an example of the very basis of managed care.

Several psychologists have maintained that exclusion from a PPO panel is essentially a "restraint of trade" in violation of the antitrust laws. In practice, however, the antitrust claims made against PPOs are often unsuccessful because managed-care businesses are typically perceived by the judiciary as being inherently procompetitive rather than anticompetitive because of their commitment to containing costs and passing the cost savings on to the consumer. Courts tend to balance the anticompetitive elements of the plan against the procompetitive ones, but the balancing test used is weighted in favor of legality. It is important to be cognizant of the fact that what may appear to be a restraint of trade is not, in itself, violative of antitrust laws. From a legal perspective, the question is whether the particular restraint of trade at issue is unreasonable and whether it places the consumer, not the provider, at a competitive disadvantage.

Courts routinely consider five factors when evaluating the reasonableness of a PPO's panel selection process. First, as was stated, courts are likely to perceive PPOs to be inherently procompetitive as opposed to anticompetitive. Second, courts acknowledge that PPOs are generally encouraged by state legislation that enables them to be established. Third, because most PPOs permit their enrollees to utilize the services of nonpreferred providers, they do not directly inhibit clinicians from practicing independently. Fourth, courts perceive PPOs as stimulating more economic choices for health care consumers. Finally, courts have typically found that because PPOs do not have a sufficiently meaningful market share, they do not completely close the marketplace to providers. These five factors combined make it difficult for an aggrieved provider to win a claim against a PPO based on antitrust grounds.

Although it is difficult to legally challenge a PPO's denial of membership to an applying psychologist, psychologists are advised to take the following steps:

- Obtain in writing the specific reasons for the refusal. One may then find it easier to devise a strategy for reapplying for panel participation.
- Determine whether the managed-care company is refusing the participation of psychologists altogether or has merely met its quota of panel psychologists. If the former situation exists, the next step is to determine whether the state's PPO law contains a willing-provider provision (15 states currently do; see APA, 1992b). Such provisions have been typically interpreted, not to guarantee panel membership to every provider who applies to a PPO panel, but rather to protect psychologists as a class of health care providers from being discriminated against and thus excluded from a panel. As a result, it is suggested that the PPO law be carefully reviewed to determine what, if any, protection exists from the particular state's insurance provision.
- Determine whether the state PPO law provides for recognition of nonpanel services. Some states require PPOs to cover the services provided by nonpreferred providers if an enrollee seeks their treatment. In such cases, the patient typically pays a higher deductible, copayment fees, or both. If the state law provides for recognition of nonpanel services and the PPO is noncompliant, the psychologist will have an excellent case to get the service in question covered.
- Determine whether the psychologist's services are delivered under a plan governed by ERISA. ERISA plans are typically not bound by state mandates.
- If no state law exists requiring that the PPO permit psychologists to serve on the panel, then the decision is usually left to the discretion of the managed-care company itself. Therefore, it is very important that the psychologist try to maintain a cordial relationship with the PPO while attempting to come to a mutually agreeable resolution. A hostile relationship will benefit no one, the patient least of all.

- If a psychologist believes that a particular PPO has a discriminatory policy against psychologists as a class, he or she should be advised to contact APA's LRA, Office of Managed Care.

No-Cause Termination

In comparison to the panel exclusion issue, the prospects for successfully challenging a no-cause termination provision appear to be gaining support as the managed-care industry evolves. It is important to keep in mind, however, that this issue has not been extensively litigated. Therefore, the information presented here represents prospective theories upon which a claim may be successfully pursued. This matter is particularly troubling for psychologists who contract with managed-care companies, because they are often placed in a position of having to negotiate with the company to allow for additional therapy sessions for their patients. There is concern, and perhaps justifiably so, that managed-care companies could arguably use the no-cause termination provision as a means of eliminating those psychologists who frequently contest decisions made by the managed-care company or its claims reviewer. This issue will be all the more critical as the number of managed-care plans increases and psychologists become increasingly dependent on managed-care companies for obtaining clients.

Several arguments can be used to challenge a managed-care company's decision to terminate a psychologist without cause. Because managed-care companies, like hospitals, have legal responsibilities, certain due process rights currently afforded to providers in a hospital setting might also be guaranteed to managed-care providers. For example, it is well established that hospitals sustain liability for failing to obtain and evaluate information regarding the training and experience of medical staff members and applicants before granting privileges. This liability also applies to managed-care companies and their credentialing procedures. Thus it has become clear that managed-care companies will have to intensify their credentialing procedures or face potential liability similar to that of hospitals (Curtis, 1990). Accordingly, it can be argued that managed-care companies, like hospitals, should be required to provide basic due process appeal rights to a provider who is terminated.

Several court cases (e.g., *Hackenthal v. California Medical Association*, 1982; *Pinsker v. Pacific Coast Society of Orthodontists*, 1969; *Salkin v. California Dental Association*, 1986) can be used to strengthen the argument for the right to appeal no-cause termination. Courts have recognized that medical professional associations and other entities related to the provision of health care are of "quasi-public" significance (Curtis, 1990); entities considered to have quasi-public significance cannot expel or discipline members, so as to adversely affect their substantial property, contract, or other economic rights, without fair proceedings. Because expulsion from a managed-care plan also involves judgment by one's own profession and such plans serve the quasi-public function of providing health care, one could argue that in no-cause termination cases, certain property and economic rights are at risk.

It can also be argued that managed-care companies have a duty to show good faith in terminating a contract. It appears that managed-care companies believe that a contract between a health care provider and a managed-care company should be treated by the courts like a standard business contract, in which no-cause termination provisions are prevalent. Although such provisions found in contracts have traditionally been held to be valid, courts have increasingly implied a duty of good faith that is intended to protect the "reasonable expectations of the parties" (Curtis, 1990). In effect, contracts with managed-care companies should be treated as agreements to provide health services rather than as simple business arrangements.

Adhesion contract theory can also be used to argue against no-cause termination. According to this theory, when a contract appears to be one-sided and unfair, particular provisions will be construed against the drafter of the contract to the extent necessary to alleviate the unfairness. Adhesion contracts are commonly found where (a) a standardized agreement is prepared by one party for the other; (b) the preparer wields superior bargaining power; and (c) the contract is offered on a take-it-or-leave-it basis, with no opportunity to bargain. These elements may be applicable to the contractual relationship between a provider and a managed-care entity in that a court may find the no-cause termination provision to be so unfair and one-sided that the provision would be void and hence unenforceable.

The following are recommended steps that can be taken by a psychologist-provider who is terminated without cause:

- Carefully review the provider contract to determine the circumstances under which a managed-care company can effectively terminate the relationship with the provider.
- If the managed-care company is able to terminate the relationship, determine whether the company has complied with the termination procedures set forth in the contract.
- To challenge a termination, upon receiving notice, contact the managed-care company's director of provider relations by phone to explore what alternatives (for redress) exist. Be as congenial as possible.
- If the telephone call is positive and feasible alternatives exist, send a written confirmation of the conversation to the managed-care company.
- In the event that the conversation with the managed-care company is negative and the provider wishes to pursue the issue further, file an official complaint with the managed-care company. Duplicate complaint letters could be sent to the state's department of insurance, which is responsible for regulating the activities of most managed-care companies.
- When appealing a termination decision in writing, the provider should cite specific reasons as to why he or she is uniquely qualified (e.g., cite a successful treatment history, a successful working relationship with the managed-care company, and additional experience or training).
- When consulting with the UR agent either to appeal a decision or to provide information to the managed-care company in support of a com-

plaint, it will be helpful to supply well-kept records and documentation of therapy.

- Be particularly sensitive to the use of the no-cause termination provision by the managed-care company as an excuse to get rid of a provider whom it may view as a troublemaker. The LRA office has received reports, based on circumstantial evidence, alleging that a psychologist was terminated from a panel merely for vigorously opposing a UR decision.

A "good plaintiff" in a no-cause-termination case is a plaintiff who has historically had a good relationship with the managed-care company but whose relationship has soured because of the plaintiff's repeated attempts to appeal or complain about a decision made by the managed-care company. Furthermore, evidence of a substantial caseload at some point during the relationship is significant, and the existence of solid documentation is essential.

Special Issues for Mental Health Professionals in Managed-Care Settings

Advantages and Disadvantages of Participating in Managed Care

Practitioners are well advised to note that the relationship between the provider and the managed-care entity is a business relationship. As a result, providers need carefully to review the managed-care plan's procedures and policies for providers in order to make a sound decision whether or not to join the entity. As was discussed previously, the two major types of managed-care entities seeking applications from psychologists are HMOs and PPOs. As in considering any business investment, psychologists should carefully weigh the advantages and disadvantages and should consider consulting an attorney before signing a contract.

There are several advantages to being a provider in a managed-care system. Managed-care entities may help to ensure an expanded patient base and more referrals for the provider. The managed-care entity will handle the marketing and the public relations of the psychologist by advertising his or her name in the benefits package. It is important to know, however, that some entities sign up a large number of participating providers but do not guarantee a particular number of patient referrals. Billing is simplified; usually payments are made directly by the managed-care company to the provider, minus the copayment. Being a member of one managed-care company may also facilitate joining others. In addition, when providers join an HMO as full-time employees, a predictable work environment may be created in which, among other advantages, they are able to benefit from affiliation with other health care providers (see chapter 8 in this book).

There are also drawbacks with managed-care arrangements. In exchange for referrals from the managed-care entity, the provider may have to agree to accept a discounted payment. The incentive for a patient to obtain services from an HMO or PPO participating provider is generally that the cost is less, and as a result, the provider can increase his or her client base by discounting fees. It has been the experience of some psychologists that an HMO or PPO will allow for coverage of only a limited number of sessions (e.g., 20 sessions per year). Frequently, services can be reduced below the covered number of sessions by the entity's UR process. Reduction of service can cause ethical and legal problems and loss of continuity of care and, at times, can result in burdensome documentation. The costs for such problems are generally absorbed by the provider. Again, it is essential for the provider to review carefully the HMO or PPO contract before signing, to ascertain, for example, whether the managed-care entity requires authorization of services in advance of treatment and whether the provider would be unable to bill the patient directly in the event that the managed-care entity disallows the payment.

Statutory and Other Protections for Practitioners

Providers should keep in mind that all states have laws to regulate HMOs. The HMO must guarantee service delivery in approved geographic areas. Any deviation by the HMO or other managed-care entity from a statutory requirement can be reported to the state department of insurance or health. The HMO laws include provisions relating to minimum benefits provided by an HMO, financial status requirements, and the composition and operation of the HMO. Likewise, many states have PPO laws and UR laws to assist the practitioner in filling regulatory complaints.

There are ways in which practitioners can protect themselves. Providers who are having difficulty obtaining participation in a managed-care entity or in resolving a complaint may wish to enlist help from a state psychological association and coordinate locally with association members. Generally, if providers join together, the managed-care entity may be more responsive. It is also important for providers to document conversations with the entity and maintain any copies of correspondence sent by or to the entity so that a written file can be accumulated.

When practitioners participate in a managed-care setting, it is important for them to become familiar with internal complaint mechanisms available to beneficiaries and providers. Before reporting a problem to the department of insurance and enlisting the help of the state and national association groups, all the remedies present within the system should be exhausted. A grievance procedure is always available, and the information about this process should be included in the documentation that is sent to both the practitioner and the beneficiary. If the information is not found in the contract, benefits package, or provider contract, then the practitioner should request copies of such materials directly from the managed-care entity. Once the practitioner has exhausted the internal grievance system, the practitioner may seek outside help by filing a complaint with the department of insurance that is responsible for regulating the particular entity involved. It is suggested that the provider contact the department of insurance to get the name of the representative who is responsible for regulating the particular entity before sending a detailed letter to the department. Copies of correspondence should also be sent to the entity involved so that it is aware that a complaint is being filed. The practitioner may also wish to send copies to the relevant professional associations to identify for the managed-care entity the level of support enlisted. However, note that a managed-care entity may drop a psychologist from membership by utilizing the termination provision set forth in the provider contract. Providers should consider this ramification when filing any complaint against a managed-care entity.

The APA Practice Directorate's *Survival Guide for the 1990s: A Marketing Handbook for Psychologists* (APA, 1992b) contains the following recommendations for evaluating a provider contract:

> One of the most critical aspects of psychology practice during the 1990s will involve negotiating fair agreements with entities seeking to contract for mental health services. It is generally recommended that practitioners consult with an attorney experienced in health care business matters to safeguard their interests and assure that all important contractual terms are covered adequately.
>
> Before seeking legal advice, psychologists can and should review proposed agreements on their own with several important questions clearly in mind, including:
>
> - Are any limitations placed on my practice prerogatives, including my ability to refer patients to providers outside the network?
> - Does the range of covered services coincide with my treatment patterns and areas of expertise?
> - Do any terms of the contracting entity's access to my client records inappropriately exceed applicable federal and state law and professional guidelines?
> - Are utilization review (UR) procedures, such as prior authorization requirements and retrospective or concurrent review, acceptable? Can I review a set of UR criteria?
> - Are any administrative requirements, such as claims filing procedures or deductible/copayment collection, unduly burdensome?
> - How are my fees paid? Do any provisions for timely payment apply to the outside entity? Can I seek payment from clients beyond covered amounts?
> - Does the contract contain a "hold-harmless" clause? Will my malpractice insurance carrier continue to cover me if I agree to such a clause? If the clause is unacceptable, will the outside entity delete it from the contract?
> - How may the contractual relationship be terminated? Would I have adequate appeal rights and a suitable mechanism for advising patients about the termination? (p. 21)

These questions are intended to help practitioners identify possible areas of concern in a proposed service contract. A good legal advisor will assist the provider in making some of the determinations prompted by the questions and with pinpointing other trouble spots in a contract.

Ethical Obligations

What are the parameters and the obligations of the psychologist providing services in a managed-care setting? When an insurance company denies a claim and a psychologist continues to treat the patient, that psychologist may assume some financial risk if he or she provides the services without guarantee of payment from the insurance company. In other words, a psychologist may not want to provide the service without guarantee of payment. If a psychologist continues to provide benefits until the appeals process is resolved, he or she should do so with the patient's understanding that the patient is responsible for charges not covered by the insurance company. Professionals should review their contract with the managed-care company to ensure that this is not a prohibited practice. Furthermore, in light of the *Wickline* (1987) and *Wilson* (1990) cases, it appears that a psychologist cannot avoid a malpractice claim simply by agreeing without protest to whatever reimbursement determination is made by the insurance company or UR entity.

Unfortunately, *Wickline* and *Wilson* really do not give us clear parameters as to how far the provider must go in terms of providing treatment to a patient whom the provider believes needs more care, but for whom the UR entity has decided further treatment is not medically necessary (Appelbaum, 1993). This specifically becomes more problematic when it is unclear whether the patient has the ability to pay. It is clear that if a provider has not begun treatment, he or she is relatively free to turn away a case, provided that the case is not an emergency. However, most UR cases center around relationships already established between the provider and the patient. A termination of this relationship creates ethical concerns for the treating psychologist. The two elements helpful for avoiding a claim of abandonment are (a) giving written notice to the patient and (b) giving the patient the opportunity to secure alternative health care services (e.g., at a community mental health center).

When UR denial applies to a truly elective procedure, there is generally ample opportunity for the provider to satisfy these two elements. However, when the patient is hospitalized or in an emergency situation, there may be no opportunity to give notice or to seek alternative treatment. In such cases, the issue of informed consent applies to the treating provider. It is important for psychologists to explain carefully to the patient, in advance of commencing treatment, the options and risks involved if the proposed treatment is denied by the UR entity. The patient must then decide whether to continue with the treatment at the risk of being held financially liable. Even if the inherent financial risk in continuing the treatment is minimal, the financial pressure on the patient makes it particularly important for the providers to explain carefully the health care risks of foregoing treatment.

Providers may believe that they are often unable to learn the basis for UR decision to deny service; however, the appeals process should provide the means of obtaining the basis for the decision. In view of the responsibility placed on the physician by *Wickline* (1987) to appeal an adverse decision, the physician should demand the basis for the UR decision on the grounds that he or she needs to respond adequately to the appeals process. Also, the UR appeals committee should prepare a written statement of its decision, which demonstrates its good-faith approach to the problem.

In advance of treatment, and as part of the informed consent process, the provider should review with the patient the proposed treatment and any procedures contractually agreed upon in the managed-care contract signed by the provider (see Bennett, Bryant, VandenBos, & Greenwood, 1990). The information provided to patients should probably outline the various contractual provisions that could affect them, including, for example, limitations on benefits, financial incentives tied to the delivery of services, and the sharing of patients' records with the managed-care entity. Providing patients with information during the initial phases of the professional relationship about the risks and limitations imposed by the real world, particularly limitations on therapeutic confidentiality, has increasingly been cited as a crucial and necessary element of psychological risk management. Section 4.02 of APA's recently revised *Ethical Principles of Psychologists and Code of Conduct* (1992a) makes the following statement about informed consent to therapy:

- Psychologists obtain appropriate informed consent to therapy or related procedures, using language that is reasonably understandable to participants. The content of informed consent will vary depending on many circumstances. However, informed consent generally implies that the person (1) has the capacity to consent, (2) has been informed of significant information concerning the procedure, (3) has freely and without undue influence expressed consent, and (4) consent has been appropriately documented.
- When persons are legally incapable of giving informed consent, psychologists obtain informed permission from a legally authorized person, if such substitute consent is permitted by law.
- In addition, psychologists (1) inform those persons who are legally incapable of giving informed consent about the proposed interventions in a manner commensurate with the person's psychological capacities, (2) seek their assent to those interventions, and (3) consider such person's preferences and best interest. (p. 1605)

At least two states now legally require informed consent as a standard of practice (Annotated Laws of Massachusetts, 1990; Oklahoma Statutes, 1991). Furthermore, there is at least anecdotal evidence that providing this information enhances, rather than diminishes, clinical effectiveness.

Informed consent is particularly important when the managed-care entity, not the psychologist or the patient, has the power to limit the reimbursement available for psychological services and may require the release of confidential information in order to determine how much treatment is warranted. Often patients have little influence over health care coverage because the coverage is provided by the employer or the employer of a spouse, and they are unaware of the limitations that the plan imposes. Mental health professionals should clarify their responsibilities to the patient and to the managed-care entity. Providers are also in the best position to notify patients of when a plan may impose limitations on coverage so that patients can investigate what those limitations are before making a decision to enter into treatment or to use their health coverage to pay for that treatment.

Mental health professionals are often confused about their responsibility to maintain the confidentiality of professionally obtained information. Their responsibility is to protect the privacy of their patients, but if their patients choose to waive that privacy, they are obligated to honor that choice. That is why the laws and ethics that govern mental health practice state that providers must maintain confidentiality unless they have the consent of their clients to do otherwise. The basic right of insurance companies to obtain information that is deemed essential to determining whether services provided are within the benefit definition (i.e., are medically necessary), is widely accepted within the insurance industry. However, private insurance carriers require patients to sign a consent form that authorizes access for the insurance company to any information that it deems appropriate to evaluating claims as a condition of coverage. Issues have been raised regarding the appropriateness and voluntariness of such consent. Many states have laws to regulate how much information an insurance company can demand and what can be done with that information. In the absence of such regulation, from a practical standpoint, releases from patients are binding, and if a patient refuses to let a practitioner submit requested information, reimbursement will be denied.

Obviously, a practitioner cannot be expected to know the details of all of the managed-care plans in the marketplace, but practitioners should be aware of the specific limitations imposed by the managed-care entity of which they are contracted members and should be prepared to discuss them with patients. The following is one example of a general information statement that a psychologist might provide to a patient in advance of treatment:

> As a licensed psychologist, the professional services I provide are usually reimbursable, in whole or in part, by insurance companies and other third-party payors. However, you should understand that although I will do my best to assist you in securing third-party reimbursement, you are responsible for payment for my services if, for any reason, such reimbursement is not available. If you belong to a managed-care plan, such as an HMO or PPO, coverage limitations are likely. If you have any questions, you should examine your plan description or contact your insurance carrier before we begin treatment. If you still have questions, I would be happy to discuss them with you.
>
> You should be aware that these third parties will often require that I provide them with information about your treatment, either in writing or over the telephone, including a clinical diagnosis and, in many cases, a treatment plan or summary. In rare cases, my entire record may be required. This information will become part of the insurance company files, and, in all probability, some of it will be computerized. All insurance carriers claim to protect the confidentiality of such information, but once it is in their hands, neither you nor I have any control over what they do with it or who may see it. Again, if you are concerned about the policies of your insurance carrier, you should check with it before authorizing me to submit the information. You have the option of paying me directly and avoiding the

creation of a record outside of this office. In the event of a specific request for information (other than that required by the claim form), I will let you know, and we can discuss the issues before I submit any information. If you wish, I will provide you with a copy of any written report that I submit.

Obviously, practitioners can edit this form so that it is consistent with their own style.

Providing information about the treatment plan and information pertaining to managed care and insurance procedures should reduce a practitioner's exposure to complaints about misconduct. First, a patient is less likely to be surprised when information is requested or when benefits for additional sessions are denied. Second, because patients are less likely to feel misled by their psychologists, psychologists are less likely to be blamed for the problems created by the managed-care coverage. Even if a patient complains about a psychologist's conduct, his or her practice of providing full information will establish that the mental health professional was behaving in a professional manner. Third, an abandonment claim would be harder to substantiate, although it obviously still would be possible, if the termination of treatment could be demonstrated to have damaged the client.

Providing this kind of information to patients may not fully satisfy a psychologist's ethical responsibility to his or her managed-care patients. Mental health professionals are also responsible for assessing whether the particular management structure is conducive to providing appropriate professional services (APA, 1992a). If the system is not appropriate, a psychologist has an ethical responsibility not to participate. If a particular plan imposes limitations on treatment, a psychologist has a responsibility to fully discuss those limitations with the patient. For example, when a managed-care plan provides reimbursement only for short-term, problem-oriented, treatment, and a psychologist feels that longer term treatment that addresses the underlying psychodynamics that have contributed to a patient's problems throughout his or her life is essential, that psychologist should discuss the costs and benefits of both short-term and long-term treatment so that the client may make a knowledgeable choice.

Furthermore, mental health professionals can provide information to patients that would enable them to advocate for their own interests with the plan manager. When an entity requests information from a provider, the patient should be informed and the request fully discussed. The patient should be reminded of the right to refuse to submit the information and to decline reimbursement. Practitioners need to be fully informed about whether relevant state law imposes any limitations on requests from insurance companies, and they should ensure that patients are aware of having access to the state's insurance commissioner if they feel aggrieved by the plan's procedures. If a patient feels that the information requested could be damaging, the provider should contact the entity and attempt to determine the necessity of such information and explore whether the information request could be satisfied in an alternative manner. Many practitioners have been successful with this approach. If the benefits manager with whom the provider speaks is nonresponsive, that provider should not hesitate to ask to speak to a supervisor.

Mental health professionals should be willing to assume a similar role when they feel that benefits are being prematurely terminated. Mental health professionals should contact the case manager to formally request and discuss the rationale for the decision to terminate treatment coverage. Providers are more likely to be effective if they can refute the entity's rationale in a measured, professional manner and less likely to be effective if they appear angry and resistant. If persuasion is not effective, the patient should be encouraged to appeal the decision, and the provider should be willing to provide assistance in that process. If benefits are terminated, there may still be a professional responsibility not to abandon the patient before making other arrangements.

References

American Psychological Association. (1992a). *Ethical principles of psychologists and code of conduct.* Washington, DC: Author.

American Psychological Association. (1992b). *Survival guide for the 1990s: A marketing handbook for psychologists.* Unpublished manuscript.

Annotated Code of Maryland—Health. (1991). 19 Md. Anno. Code Sec. 116.

Annotated Laws of Massachusetts. (1981). Mass. Anno. Laws ch. 176A, Sec. 10A. Eagan, MN: West.

Annotated Laws of Massachusetts. (1990). Mass. Anno. Laws Ch. 13, Sec. 129A.

Annotated Statutes of Minnesota. (1986). Minn. Anno. Stat. 72A.20(15)(4). Eagan, MN: West.

Appelbaum, P. S. (1993). Legal Liability and Managed Care. *American Psychologist, 48*, 251–257.

Arkansas Code Annotated. (1987). 23 Ark. Code Anno. Secs. 76–101 et seq., 98–109. Charlottesville, VA: Michie.

Becker, J., Tiano, L., & Marshall, S. (1992). Legal issues in managed mental health. In R. Fitzpatrick & J. L. Feldman (Eds.), *Managed Mental Health Care: Administration and clinical issues* (pp. 6–8). Washington, DC: American Psychiatric Press.

Bennett, B. E., Bryant, B. K., VandenBos, G. R., & Greenwood, A. (1990). *Professional liability and risk management.* Washington, DC: American Psychological Association.

Black, H. C. (1979). *Black's law dictionary.* St. Paul, MN: West.

Boochever, S. (1986). Health maintenance organizations. In J. M. Johnson (Ed.), *Introduction to alternative delivery mechanisms: HMOs, PPOs & CMPs* (pp. 5–10). Washington, DC: National Health Lawyers Association.

Boyd v. Albert Einstein Medical Center, 547 A.2d 1229 (Pa. Super. Ct. 1988).

Brodman, S. F. (1993, August 3). The White House is banking on HMOs as a way to reform health care but many HMOs skimp on health care benefits. *The Washington Post* (Health Section), p. 11.

Corcoran v. United Health Care, 965 F.2d 1321 (5th cir. 1992).

Curtis, T. (1990). Fair hearings for physicians denied participation in managed care plans. *Medical Staff Counselor, 4*, 45–47.

Dickstein, D., Hanig, D., & Grosskopf, B. (1988). Reducing treatment costs in a community support program. *Hospital and Community Psychiatry, 39*, 1033–1035.

District of Columbia Code Annotated, Section 35-2310 (1993).

Employee Retirement Income Security Act of 1974. 29 U.S.C. Section 1142 (1982).

Georgia Code Annotated, §§ 33-21-1 [et seq., 45-1] (1990). Charlottesville, VA: Michie.

Hackenthal v. California Medical Association, 187 Cal. Rptr. 811 (Ct. App. 1982).

Harbaugh, C. (1993, February). Courts All Over the Map on Plan Liability for Allegedly Negligent Actions of Physicians. *Managed Care Law Outlook, 5*(2), 10–11.

Harrell v. Total Health Care, Inc., 781 S.W.2d 58 (Mo. 1989).

Health Maintenance Organization Act of 1973, Section 280(c), 300(e)(1)(b), 300(e)(1)(c)–(6)(a), 300(e)(1)(d), 42 U.S.C. (1987).

Hinden, R. A., & Elden, D. L. (1990). Liability issues for managed care entities. *Seton Hall Legislative Journal, 14*(8), 1–60.

Hughs v. Blue Cross of Northern California, 215 Cal. App. 3d 832, Cal. Ct. App. (1989).

Illinois Revised Statutes. (1986). Ill. Rev. Stat. ch. 73, para 982h, Eagan, MN: Smith-Hurd Supp. 806.

Kentucky Administrative Regulations. (1991). Ky. Admin. Regs. 18:020.

McClellan v. Health Maintenance Organization of Pennsylvania. 604 A. 2nd 1053 (Pa. Super. Ct. 1992).

Michigan Compiled Laws Annotated. (1988). Mich. Comp. Laws Anno. Secs. 14.15 et seq., 24.650(56). Eagan, MN: West.

National Association of Insurance Commissioners. (1989). Model Health Maintenance Organization Act. Washington, DC: Author.

Nebraska Revised Statutes. (1987). Neb. Rev. Stat. Sec. 44, 44-409.

Oklahoma Statutes. (1991). Okla. Stat. tit. 59, Sec. 1376.

Pinsker v. Pacific Coast Society of Orthodontists, 460 P.2d 495 (Cal. 1969).

Revised Statutes Annotated of Arizona. (1992). Secs. 20–1051. Charlottesville, VA: Michie.

Salkin v. California Dental Association, 224 Cal Rptr. 352 (Ct. App. 1986).

Salley v. E. D. DuPont de Nemours & Company, No. 91-35-23 (5th Cir. 1992).

Schleier v. Kaiser Foundation Health Plan, 876 F.2d 174 (D.C. Cir. 1989).

Sloan v. Metropolitan Health Council of Indianapolis, Inc., 516 N.E. 2d 1104 (Ind. Ct. App. 1987).

Steele, C. J. (1992, September). Court says ERISA pre-empts benefit-denial claims of malpractice against covered plans. *Managed Care Law Outlook, 4*(9), 2–6.

Tax Equity and Fiscal Responsibility Act of 1982, 42 U.S.C. Section 1395 (1987).

Wickline v. State of California, 239 Cal. Rptr. 805, 741 P.2d 613 (1987).

Wilson v. Blue Cross of Southern California, 271 Cal. Rptr. 876, Cal. App. 2 Dist. (1990).

6

Mental Health Claims Experience: Analysis and Benefit Redesign

Rodney L. Lowman

As employers and third-party insurers seek ways to contain mental health costs, a major and rather neglected area for fast-acting and potentially long-lasting cost relief is the analysis of mental health claims experience and, where appropriate, the redesign of mental health benefits. Through detailed study of the actual mental health utilization experience of covered populations, mental health payers can determine how their mental health dollars are being spent, whether cost problems exist, and the specific areas to which cost-containment efforts may best be directed. Such analyses can also enable third-party payers to track over time whether cost-containment efforts are affecting use and payment patterns. The value of mental health claims analysis as an important management tool for cost containment and quality assurance is illustrated with claims data from one large employer.

A second, related focus of this chapter is on mental health benefit redesign. Clearly, the fastest and most long-lasting way to contain mental health costs is simply to cut drastically the mental health benefit offered by indemnity or health maintenance organization (HMO) plans. This chapter demonstrates that the typical mental health benefit plan is designed—I assume unintentionally—to encourage the use of more costly treatment modalities by penalizing those who use less expensive but often equally or more effective treatment approaches. As demonstrated in this chapter, mental health benefits can be redesigned to reflect both what is known about the claims experiences of a covered population and current literature findings on the relative efficacy of various treatment methods.

Mental Health Benefit Claims Analysis

A Case Study in Mental Health Benefit Analysis

Illustrative of the process and value of mental health benefit claims analysis are the multiyear data provided by Company X. Although the name of this

Reprinted from *Professional Psychology: Research and Practice, 22*, 36–44. (1991). Copyright 1991 by the American Psychological Association.

Table 1. Annual Health and Mental Health Expenditures
(in U.S. Dollars) of Company X, 1987–1989

Costs	1987	1988	1989
Combined health & mental health			
Inpatient	3,511,783	4,160,934	4,286,247
Outpatient	1,907,088	2,316,135	2,868,835
Total	5,418,871	6,477,069	7,155,082
Mental health			
Substance abuse	56,041	108,586	49,122
Mental & nervous	363,172	460,071	418,581
Total	419,213	568,657	467,703
Mental health as percentage of total health care	7.7%	8.8%	6.5%

employer and its insurance company have been withheld by request of the client organization, it can be noted that the covered population included about 1,800 employees, mostly men, and their family members (mostly women and children). As is typical of many mental health benefit plans, this company covered the costs of mental health inpatient services the same as for any other illness (including up to 150 days of hospital care). However, outpatient care was covered on only a 50% basis (i.e., after deductibles, the plan paid for only 50% of the costs of outpatient mental health care, up to a defined dollar limit). The data presented in this chapter cover a 2.5–3-year period, offering the unusual feature of allowing cross-year tracking of mental health services consumed by individual users.

Table 1 shows the total health care expenditures for the client company through the benefit plan for calendar years 1987, 1988, and 1989.

As Table 1 indicates, direct overall company expenditures[1] on health care rose by $1,058,198 from 1987 to 1988, and by $510,791 from 1988 to 1989, demonstrating typical 15.8% and 5.8% respective increases (see Broskowski, chapter 1 in this book). Expenditures for substance abuse rose by 94.2% between 1987 and 1988, declining in 1989 by 54.8% over the record high 1988 figures. Total mental health (substance abuse and nervous and mental costs) rose by 57% from 1987 to 1988. As a percentage of total health care expenditures, mental health costs rose from 7.7% in 1987 to 8.8% in 1988 and declined to 6.5% in 1989.

Table 2 breaks down the overall health costs (mental and nonmental) for 1987, 1988, and 1989 into inpatient and outpatient care by age and category of user. In 1987, 65% of the company's overall health care costs went for

---

[1]All data are based on the employer's expenditures and exclude employees' copayment and deductibles, which are not tracked by the company. These figures also do not take into account subtractions for Medicare and coordination of benefits with other carriers. Thus, although the figures reflect total plan liability, the actual amounts paid out by the insurance administrator were slightly lower than the figures summarized here, and the total costs expended from all sources would be slightly higher.

Table 2.   Overall Medical Costs (in U.S. Dollars) by Age and Category of Use

Age	Inpatient	%	Outpatient	%	Total	%
			1987			
0–24	658,495	18.8	377,836	19.8	1,036,331	19.1
25–34	388,942	11.1	222,237	11.7	611,179	11.3
35–44	394,077	11.2	261,538	13.7	655,615	12.1
45–54	865,653	24.6	472,708	24.8	1,338,361	24.7
55–64	1,003,118	28.6	468,849	24.6	1,471,967	27.2
65–74	197,627	5.6	100,046	5.2	297,673	5.5
Over 75	3,871	0.1	3,874	0.2	7,745	0.1
Total	3,511,783	100	1,907,088	100	5,418,871	100
			1988			
0–24	778,415	18.7	432,514	18.7	1,210,929	18.7
25–34	427,637	10.3	235,331	10.2	662,968	10.2
35–44	510,386	12.3	341,661	14.8	852,047	13.2
45–54	798,371	19.2	531,869	23.0	1,330,240	20.5
55–64	1,107,504	26.6	611,316	26.4	1,718,820	26.5
65–74	502,386	12.1	159,074	6.9	661,460	10.2
Over 75	36,235	0.9	4,370	0.2	40,605	0.6
Total	4,160,934	100	2,316,135	100	6,477,069	100
			1989			
0–24	619,132	14.4	531,816	18.5	1,150,948	16.1
25–34	360,577	8.4	299,040	10.4	659,617	9.2
35–44	505,542	11.8	387,934	13.5	893,476	12.5
45–54	902,003	21.0	606,357	21.1	1,508,360	21.1
55–64	1,235,957	28.8	803,612	28.0	2,039,569	28.5
65–74	657,115	15.3	235,529	8.2	892,644	12.5
Over 75	5,921	0.1	4,547	0.2	10,468	0.1
Total	4,286,247	100	2,868,835	100	7,155,082	100

inpatient care, 64% in 1988, and 60% in 1989. By examining the age distribution of users of mental health services, one can see that about one half of the overall expenditures in all 3 years went to the care of persons in the 45–64-year age bracket, consistent with the expected increase of medical problems with increasing age. These figures also express the demographics of the company's work force, which is characterized by considerable seniority.

However, although the overall medical costs reflect relative balance in the inpatient–outpatient breakdown and a predictable age utilization curve favoring older persons in the sample, a different pattern is presented by the nervous and mental health costs (see Table 3). In this case, 94% of costs in 1987 and 1988 and 91% in 1989 were for inpatient care. Comparable figures at the national level show around 70% to 75% of mental health costs being expended on inpatient care (Lowman, 1987; Mosher, 1983). Table 3 shows that more than half of the inpatient costs of mental and nervous care and of substance abuse care for 1987 and 1988 and about 47% for 1989 went for services provided to individuals in the 0–24-year and 25–34-year age brackets. The 55–64-year group was also a comparatively high inpatient use group.

Table 3. Nervous and Mental Health Costs (in U.S. Dollars) and Substance Abuse Costs (in U.S. Dollars) by Age and Category of Use

Age	Inpatient	%	Outpatient	%	Total	%
			1987			
0–24	138,308	35.2	6,356	23.8	144,664	34.5
25–34	101,048	25.7	2,537	9.5	103,585	24.7
35–44	24,434	6.2	4,870	18.2	29,304	7.0
45–54	25,937	6.6	6,190	23.2	32,127	7.7
55–64	102,798	26.2	6,717	25.2	109,515	26.1
65–74	0	0	19	0.0	19	0
Over 75	0	0	0	0.0	0	0
Total	392,525	100	26,689	100	419,214	100
			1988			
0–24	178,832	33.5	8,002	23.0	186,834	32.9
25–34	89,996	16.9	4,899	14.1	94,895	16.7
35–44	116,239	21.8	8,797	25.2	125,036	22.0
45–54	23,883	4.5	6,098	17.5	29,981	5.3
55–64	113,648	21.3	6,019	17.3	119,667	21.0
65–74	11,197	2.1	1,047	3.0	12,244	2.2
Over 75	0	0	0	0.0	0	0
Total	533,795	100	34,862	100	568,657	100
			1989			
0–24	191,840	45.0	7,430	18.1	199,270	42.6
25–34	16,772	4.0	4,492	10.9	21,264	4.5
35–44	132,220	31.0	9,411	22.9	141,631	30.3
45–54	22,734	5.3	6,427	15.6	29,161	6.2
55–64	32,744	7.7	12,651	31.0	45,395	9.7
65–74	30,285	7.1	697	1.7	30,982	6.6
Over 75	0	0	0	0	0	0
Total	426,595	100	41,108	100	467,703	100

Tables 4 and 5 show nervous and mental and substance abuse costs by sex, category of use (inpatient vs. outpatient), and category of user (employee, spouse, child–adolescent dependent). These figures exemplify the need to examine demographic-specific cost utilization data in conducting mental health claims analysis.

Several trends are evident in the category of user of mental health care treatment (Table 4). Contrary to the medical utilization patterns noted above, for mental and nervous care a large amount was spent for the care of dependent children, especially for care provided in inpatient treatment units. Until 1989, substance abuse costs were primarily incurred by employees and dependents; however, in that year the largest expenditure was for dependent children, which suggests a possible area for attention and programmatic intervention efforts by the employer or third-party payer. These patterns reflect national trends (see Weithorn, 1988, for an excellent review). Company X spent $469,398 for the mental health care of dependent children over the 3-year period. For the child and adolescent group, an average of 99% of this cost was for inpatient

Table 4. Mental and Nervous Treatment Costs (in U.S. Dollars) by Sex and Category of User

User	1987			1988			1989		
	Inpatient	Outpatient	Total	Inpatient	Outpatient	Total	Inpatient	Outpatient	Total
Employees									
Male	78,761	6,874	85,635	173,226	9,783	183,009	121,423	12,404	133,827
Female	18,751	1,993	20,744	3,409	1,591	5,000	0	2,073	2,073
Total	97,512	8,867	106,379	176,635	11,374	188,009	121,423	14,477	135,900
Spouses									
Male	0	0	0	54	252	306	(54)[a]	0	(54)
Female	83,964	10,495	94,459	84,743	13,823	98,566	129,966	18,896	148,862
Total	83,964	10,495	94,459	84,797	14,075	98,872	129,912	18,896	148,808
Dependent children									
Male	56,260	4,706	60,966	153,780	4,880	158,660	77,292	4,767	82,059
Female	99,521	1,848	101,369	11,376	3,154	14,530	50,069	1,745	51,814
Total	155,781	6,554	162,335	165,156	8,034	173,190	127,361	6,512	133,873
All users	337,257	25,916	363,173	426,588	33,483	460,071	378,696	39,885	418,581

Note. Excludes substance abuse.
[a]Credit in original.

Table 5. Substance Abuse Treatment Costs (in U.S. Dollars) by Sex and Category of User

User	1987			1988			1989		
	Inpatient	Outpatient	Total	Inpatient	Outpatient	Total	Inpatient	Outpatient	Total
Employees									
Male	43,645	676	44,321	66,737	303	67,040	4,991	0	4,991
Female	0	98	98	728	265	993	0	899	899
Total	43,645	774	44,419	67,465	568	68,033	4,991	899	5,890
Spouses									
Male	0	0	0	0	0	0	0	0	0
Female	11,622	0	11,622	25,610	769	26,379	0	250	250
Total	11,622	0	11,622	25,610	769	26,379	0	250	250
Dependent children									
Male	0	0	0	14,134	40	14,174	25,910	42	25,952
Female	0	0	0	0	0	0	17,000	30	17,030
Total	0	0	0	14,134	40	14,174	42,910	72	42,982
All users	55,267	774	56,041	107,209	1,377	108,586	47,901	1,221	49,122

care in 1988 and 1989. Whereas men were the principal employee users of mental health care (consistent with the sex demographics of the work force) and women were the principal spouse users, there was more variability in the dependent children group, with both boys and girls incurring large charges.

Individual Patterns of Utilization of Mental Health Services

Grouped data are valuable for identifying trends in overall costs and utilization of medical and mental health services, but they tend to mask important individual-level cost and utilization patterns. Typically, in mental health services (and possibly in medical services as well), it is a relatively small number of users who account for large dollar amounts of services (Broskowski, chapter 1).

Unfortunately, because of artifacts of the data collection system, individ-

Table 6. Number and Cost (in U.S. Dollars) of Mental Health Claims by Selected Periods

Group	1987	1988	January–June 1989
Employees			
No. of claims	63	63	44
Cost	128,880	222,273	47,261
Average cost per claim	2,046	3,528	1,074
Spouses			
No. of claims	44	67	44
Cost	106,066	109,657	105,720
Average cost per claim	2,411	1,637	2,403
Dependent children			
No. of claims	31	28	27
Cost	146,967	112,119	77,490
Average cost per claim	4,741	4,004	2,870
Totals			
No. of claims	138	158	115
Cost	381,913	444,049	230,471
Average cost per claim	2,767	2,810	2,004

Table 7. Number of Patients Filing Claims Across More Than 1 Year

Patients	1988: Repeats from 1987	1989: Repeats from 1987	1989: Repeats from 1988
Employees	24	10	21
Spouses	17	8	22
Children	10	7	8
Total	51	25	52

Note. Five of the children, eight of the spouses, and eight of the employees were represented across all three of the periods presented in the study.

Table 8. Costs (in U.S. Dollars) of Multiple Year Consumers of Mental Health Services, Child and Adolescent Cases

Case	1987	1988	January–June, 1989	Total
1	34,041	36,882	37	70,960
2	18	19	115	152
3	600	363	265	1,228
4	109	458		567
5	210	649		859
6	448		8,713	9,161
7	5,393	16,913		22,306
8	2	5,452		5,454
9	310	70	395	775
10	340		89	429
11	739	208		947
12		2,125	13,774	15,899
13		735	48	783
14		6,572	40	6,612
15	2,339	81	259	2,679
Total	44,549	70,527	23,735	138,811

Unfortunately, because of artifacts of the data collection system, individual-level analyses were not possible with the data so far presented. The design of the data collection system did not even allow the determination of the number of individual cases represented in each category because the unit of analysis was the number of claims filed rather than number of individuals served. Moreover, these data were generated on the basis of the date that claims were processed rather than the date that the care was rendered.

For the individual-level analyses, it was therefore necessary to have the insurance carrier compute new statistics, which in this case necessitated using a slightly different data base, to permit individual claims to be analyzed. (Note that, because the data base differs, the summary statistics for these analyses do not correspond to the totals from the previously presented data; therefore, the totals should not be compared. Also, for these analyses, only half-year data from 1989 were available.)

Statistics on the costs of care that was rendered in each of the three periods under study are presented in Table 6. The data include any claims resulting in a cost to the insurance plan of more than $1.00. Only 63 cases (i.e., separate individuals) were represented in the 1987 and 1988 analyses, and 44 were included in the 1989 half-year data.

Employee populations for the 1987, 1988, and 1989 periods were 1,734, 1,756, and 1,795, respectively. Using an estimated average of one spouse per individual employee and 1.5 children per family (2,601, 2,634, and 2,693 child dependents per year, respectively), the total covered population for the three periods would be 6,069, 6,146, and 6,283, respectively. These figures are slightly higher than the actual number of covered individuals because the employee figures include new employees not covered by the indemnity plan at the time of their initial employment, although the company did little new hiring during the covered period.

Table 9. Costs (in U.S. Dollars) of Multiple Year Consumers of Mental Health Services, Spouse Cases

Case	1987	1988	January–June, 1989	Total
1	174	1,504		1,678
2		10	333	343
3		413	60	473
4		518	96	614
5	524	2,278		2,802
6	392	134		526
7	2,488	29		2,517
8	6,878	324	94	7,296
9	105	195		300
10	80	16,882	15,819	32,781
11		385	105	490
12		51	27	78
13		1,402	735	2,137
14		109	243	352
15		110	46,521	46,631
16	2,891	270		3,161
17	80	368	475	923
18	58	25		83
19	240	596	12,895	13,731
20	603	285	415	1,303
21	227	103		330
22		125	176	301
23		31	42	73
24	284	443	413	1,140
25	1,590	262	85	1,937
26	775	702		1,477
27	44,878	39,757	13	84,648
28		9,807	446	10,253
29		260	35	295
30		50	64	114
31		24	17	41
Total	62,267	77,452	79,109	218,828

Comparison of the estimated covered population data with the utilization data presented in Table 6 shows that, on average, about 2.3%, 2.6%, and (for the half year 1989) 1.8% of the estimated covered population used mental health services. Although this fraction of individuals is rather small, the costs of services rendered are not, as the average claim summarized in Table 6 demonstrates.

As years are an artificial boundary for grouping mental health claims data, I examined individual-level data for the 2½-year period discussed here, to determine whether the same individuals were responsible for large mental health claims year after year. Table 7 shows the number of individuals who filed claims during more than one period of the covered years. This table summarizes the number of repeat cases from 1987 to 1988, from 1987 to the first half of 1989, and from 1988 to the first half of 1989.

The dollar values associated with these cases are examined next. Tables

Table 10. Costs (in U.S. Dollars) of Multiple Year Consumers of Mental Health Services,Employee Cases

Case	1987	1988	January–June 1989	Total
1	4,665	1,920		6,585
2	18,936	4,015		22,951
3	821		285	1,106
4	40	794	300	1,134
5	11,487	50		11,537
6	4,696	5,960		10,656
7	13,422	29,190		42,612
8		10	16	26
9		65	48	113
10		45	110	155
11		27,148	6,753	33,901
12	18	255		273
13	18	102		120
14	165	789		954
15	847	643	385	1,875
16		25,484	16,510	41,994
17		11,985	14	11,999
18		7,079	895	7,974
19	356	20,498		20,854
20	4,469	1,225		5,694
21	1,616	59	34	1,709
22	39	17		56
23	325	273	31	629
24	16	156	100	272
25	405	7,468	453	8,326
26	9,877	519		10,396
27	590	541		1,131
28	80	357		437
29	5,176	46,379		51,555
30	22,413	679	36	23,128
31	342	365	425	1,132
32	338	25		363
33	80		77	157
34		38,611	696	39,307
35		1,666	60	1,726
36		15	58	73
37		72	17	89
38		202	14	216
39		366	366	732
Total	101,237	235,027	27,683	363,947

8, 9, and 10 present the intriguing results of the costs of the cases from Table 7 (i.e., those having claims in more than one of the examined periods). Although these cases are few in number compared with the covered population, they account for a very large portion of the expended mental health insurance benefits. For the child and adolescent cases (Table 8), only 5 of the 15 cases

(Numbers 1, 6, 7, 12, and 14) incurred a combined cost to the plan of $124,938, or 90% of the repeated-cases total. Note that more than half (51%) of the total cost of these cases is accounted for by Case 1 alone and that this individual had the highest claims filed in *both* 1987 and 1988.

A similar pattern emerges for both the spouse and employee groups (Tables 9 and 10, respectively). For the spouses (Table 9), the five most expensive cases (Numbers 10, 15, 19, 27, and 28) cost a total of $180,044, or 86% of the total. For employees (Table 10), the five most expensive cases (Numbers 7, 11, 16, 29, and 34) cost $209,369, or 58% of the total during the 2½-year period. (Although this percentage is lower than those of the other two groups, the number of cases of cross-year treatment is larger.)

Clearly, in the case of this organization, mental health benefits claims include several areas of potentially problematic mental health benefit utilization. However, the number of affected individuals is actually quite small, so that efforts may need to be directed in this case more to case management than to population-wide prevention. Further data on diagnosis and types of problems incurred by the affected individuals, especially the high-dollar users, would enable a more targeted cost-containment effort (possibly in conjunction with the company's employee assistance program) to be developed.

Implications for Mental Health Claims Analysis

Obtaining and analyzing the data reported in this article required considerable effort and expense. However, the utility of these data for managing mental health costs can readily be seen. Claims experience data are useful to a company both retrospectively, when it seeks to understand where and how its insurance money has been expended, and also concurrently, when it is still possible to contain problematic costs.

Consistent with the analyses presented here, the following data are recommended for routine collection and monitoring in evaluating the claims experiences of particular employers or insurance companies:

1. *Costs for mental health treatment through the indemnity or other insurance plan.* Overall costs for health and mental health care need to be monitored on a regular basis, preferably at least semiannually if control over the costs is to be obtained. Analyses should minimally include (a) absolute dollars expended on mental health care; (b) costs as a percentage of total health care expenditures; (c) inpatient versus outpatient mental health costs; (d) substance abuse versus other mental health treatment costs; and (e) costs with and without the costs of any employee assistance program.

2. *Number and demographics of covered individuals treated.* Because different mental health consumption patterns would be expected depending on the demographic makeup of the insured population, costs should be analyzed by the following categories: (a) *type of users*: employees, adult dependents, and adolescent and child dependents as consumers of mental health services; (b) *demographics of users*: age, sex, and employee status of the various consumers of insured mental health services; (c) *one-time versus ongoing users*: cross-year

users should be tracked on an ongoing basis; and (d) *family unit*: if possible, the mental health consumption of services by members of the same family should be analyzed to determine familial usage and the possible influence of psychological distress on multiple members of the same family. It should be emphasized that individual-level data should be analyzed only in a manner that protects the identity of the individuals receiving mental health services or in which the analyses are conducted by a trained mental health professional bound by professional ethics to rules of confidentiality.

3. *Average length of inpatient stay:* Tracking of average lengths of stay should ideally occur on an interactive rather than retrospective basis. Because inpatient care is so costly, special efforts must be directed to the containment of its costs. In a prospective control system, patients are monitored as to utilization of inpatient care before they reach the hospital, and a case management system might be used in the effort to reduce costs. At a minimum, employers and insurance companies need to compute the number of inpatient days by various categories of patients and, if possible, the differential utilization of hospital days by provider. In addition, where possible, data should be analyzed (a) by facility providing care; (b) by substance abuse versus other types of mental health care; (c) by diagnosis of case; (d) for each of these categories, by the groupings of employees, spouses, and child and adolescent dependents. Each of these data analyses have action steps that can be taken if the associated usage of mental health services is excessive.

4. *Diagnostic category:* Both direct and indirect costs associated with all psychiatric and substance abuse disorders should be tracked, regardless of where the mental health services might be delivered. Costs associated with patients who have underlying psychiatric disorders and who are treated within medical facilities may not show up with current analytical methods. Patients hospitalized in a medical unit for treatment of medical problems secondary to chronic alcohol abuse may not appear in the substance abuse summary statistics for the overall costs of substance abuse care. Ideally, cost analyses can also be done for conditions in which mental health diagnoses are secondary rather than primary.

Implications for Mental Health Benefit Redesign

The case example provides a method for pinpointing the source of cost problems in typical data sets and also illustrates that the same individuals may be recurrent high utilizers of mental health services. What, then, can be done to improve the situation?

Extreme problems may call for extreme solutions. By far the easiest solution to the present dilemma is simply to redesign mental health benefits to encourage a more judicious use of services and to put limits on the dollars consumed by those most inclined to generate large costs. Where allowed by state laws or other guidelines, employers and insurance companies might drastically limit the mental health benefit, particularly for the more expensive and less proved inpatient treatment modalities.

However, there are strong arguments to be made against this approach. Untreated substance abuse problems, for example, are associated with high costs of medical care and with increased medical costs of nonabusing family members. Moreover, studies have persistently demonstrated the efficacy of treating psychological problems and the shortsightedness of cutting mental health benefits. (The costs of physical treatment care go up when this happens.) Furthermore, by analogy, although a small percentage of people benefit from medical services for serious illnesses (e.g., for myocardial infarction or onco- logical services), few would argue for eliminating treatment of cancer or car- diologic problems simply because a small part of an insured population needs the service. Moreover, in some states such actions would be illegal (see Newman & Bricklin, chapter 4 in this book).

In most states, however, the mental health benefit could be significantly lowered without violating legal mandates. Although such a severe course might immediately lower mental health costs, the long-range consequences might be severe. Ideally, mental health benefit design would be based on a rationale and an empirical research base that optimize the trade-off between cost con- tainment and quality control, and not merely mimic tradition inherited from medical insurance benefit design. Presumably, employers do not want to cut off services from those in need, but neither do they wish to make excessive expenditures; the design should reflect this goal.

If blanket benefit curtailment is not the answer, are there any effective ways for decreasing mental health costs? One clue is provided in a persistent and often overlooked factor, illustrated by the data presented in this article: Generally, a small minority of employees and their family members make use of mental health services, and among such users, a small number of cases can account for the largest amount of expense for the company. Rather than making mental health benefits unavailable to those in need, a better solution would be tighter control of the high-cost cases, generally few in number but often extremely expensive to treat.

Because numerous studies (see Goldstein & Horgan, 1988), including the present one, have demonstrated that mental health *inpatient* costs currently account for the bulk of the expenditures, they are the costs that need most control. However, consideration must also be directed to the liberalization of outpatient costs, which are typically second class compared with inpatient benefits. This long-standing policy of favoring inpatient care has provided an inherent incentive for the use of the most costly treatment alternatives to deal with serious mental health problems.

Efficacy of Inpatient Care Versus Outpatient Alternatives

A critical question in designing mental health benefits is the relative efficacy of the care to be paid for through the plan. If inpatient care is demonstrated to result in outcomes superior to outpatient alternatives, then it may be ap- propriate for mental health benefits to be designed in a manner that rewards the use of inpatient care. If, however, inpatient care is not demonstrated to be a treatment of choice for the seriously psychologically impaired, then a case can be made for making that care more difficult to obtain than outpatient alternatives.

Space does not permit a detailed exploration of the literature on outcomes of inpatient mental health care. (For a more detailed review see Kiesler, 1982; Lowman, 1987; Parker & Knoll, 1990.) However, although there is need for further study of the issue, inpatient care has generally not fared well when compared with outpatient alternatives. The literature has generally demonstrated that hospital treatment of the psychologically impaired has rarely shown superior results to outpatient alternatives (e.g., Hayashida et al., 1989; Kiesler, 1982; Langsley, Flomenhaft, & Machotka, 1969; Langsley & Kaplan, 1969; Langsley, Pittman, Machotka, & Flomenhaft, 1968; Mosher, 1983; Mosher & Menn, 1978; Pasamanick, Scarpitti, & Dinitz, 1967; Weithorn, 1988); and that, among patients who are hospitalized for psychiatric impairments, long-term stays generally do not result in outcomes superior to short-term stays (Braun et al., 1981; Endicott, Cohen, Nee, Fleiss, & Herz, 1979; Glick, Hargreaves, & Goldfield, 1974; Gordon & Breakey, 1983; Herz, Endicott, & Gibbon, 1979; Herz, Endicott, & Spitzer, 1975; Kirshner, 1982; Mattes, Rosen, & Klein, 1977; Weisman, Feinstein, & Thomas, 1969). The data are somewhat more limited for nonadult cases, but these general findings appear to apply to children and adolescents as well as to adults (e.g., Amini, Zilberg, Burke, & Salasnek, 1982; Blotcky, Dimperio, & Gossett, 1984; Rosenstock, 1985), although the literature is somewhat less extensive. Yet mental health benefits are generally designed as if exactly the opposite were true. Such plans all too typically reimburse for inpatient care more generously than for outpatient alternatives and, in many but not all cases, reimburse for long-term hospital stays at a rate higher than for short-term stays (in that major medical plans may pay more for the longer term care). In both cases, a perverse incentive is provided to use more costly and seemingly less effective treatment modalities. The situation appears to be particularly acute among children and youth, who presumably have less control over the type or length of their care (see Knitzer, 1982; Lowman, 1987; Melton, in press; Milasso-Sayre, Benson, Rosestein, & Manderscheid, 1986; Weithorn, 1988). Recent data suggest that the same conclusions may apply to substance abuse, another high-cost item in the typical insurance plan. Hayashida et al. (1989), for example, randomly assigned patients to outpatient and inpatient detoxification treatment protocols. These patients were male veterans of low socioeconomic status. Outpatient cases were detoxified in an average of 6.5 days, compared with 9.2 days for inpatients, although more individuals in the inpatient than in the outpatient condition completed the detoxification program. At the 6-month follow-up period there was no difference between the two groups in substance abuse-related problems, medical problems, or need for further treatment. However, the cost for treating inpatients was significantly higher (more than $3,000 per inpatient treatment versus less than $400 for outpatient treatment). Certainly it would be inappropriate to generalize from the results of one study, but this important work lends credence to the view that, as with mental health problems, substance abuse may effectively be treated in outpatient settings.

Typical Mental Health Benefit Design

Mental health benefits appear largely to be based on the design of traditional medical benefit plans. Typically, inpatient care is paid for by third-party payers at the rate of 80% of the costs (the typical 80–20 design, although sometimes 100% is covered), whereas 50% of outpatient care is reimbursed. Often outpatient care has a very low per-session dollar allowance, so that a small fraction of the costs of the care are paid by the third party. Outpatient alternatives to inpatient care (e.g., day hospitals or family crisis programs) are often reimbursed as regular outpatient care at a very low rate.

The reasoning in this design appears to have been that the burden of costly inpatient care should be borne by distributing risk across a larger population, whereas the presumably more inexpensive outpatient care could be shouldered more readily by individuals receiving the treatment. In the instance of mental health, however, assumptions about the efficacy of inpatient care for serious mental health problems must be questioned. Studies that have examined the efficacy of inpatient care versus outpatient alternatives for psychological dysfunctions have generally shown that the two treatment types are at least equal in effectiveness, or more typically, that outpatient care results in a superior outcome, generally at considerably lower cost than inpatient alternatives. The typical mental health benefit design is therefore inconsistent with literature findings on treatment effectiveness.

Because behavior is at least partially the consequence of incentives, current benefit plans that favor inpatient care at the expense of outpatient care result in the predictable outcome that inpatient care rather than outpatient care is used when the insured have a choice. Mental health management systems that can reject or cut the length of inpatient treatment but cannot make outpatient treatment programs more accessible would be expected to have little effect on overall cost containment. A benefit plan that follows the current literature would liberally cover the costs of reasonable lengths of outpatient care (at least for conditions with a demonstrated track record of responding to outpatient care) and place firm limits on the amount of inpatient care covered. Were form to follow function in benefit design, if the goal is clinically effective, cost-contained treatment, then inpatient care would be limited and outpatient care would be made much more accessible (see Kiesler, 1982; Mosher, 1983; Parloff, 1982).

Alternatives to Traditional Mental Health Benefit Design

Of course there is nothing magical or preordained about how mental health benefits are designed, just as the 80–20 split so commonly found in mental health benefit plans is not mandated by any authority other than tradition. Alternative benefit designs can be developed to encourage the use of less costly treatment modalities. Table 11 illustrates an alternative benefit design.

In this model, inpatient care is deemphasized and outpatient care is encouraged. To emphasize short-term care (to which most psychological problems are responsive), a graduated copayment can be introduced. Similarly, short-

Table 11. Illustrative Revised Health Benefit Plan

Utilization	Percentage paid by third party	Percentage paid by patient
Outpatient		
First 10 visits	100	0
Next 10 visits	75	25
Next 10 visits	50	50
Next 10 visits	25	75
After 40 visits	0	100
Day hospital—other outpatient intensive		
First 30 days	80	20
Next 15 days	50	50
Next 15 days	20	80
After 60 days	0	100
Inpatient		
First 5 days	90	10
Next 15 days	70	30
Next 15 days	50	50
After 25 days	0	100

term outpatient care would be highly reimbursed, and long-term care (for which the efficacy is less proved) would require a higher deductible. On the other hand, the goal is not simply to change an apparent cost problem from inpatient to outpatient care; therefore, limits on what is paid for in outpatient care must also be considered.

Summary and Conclusions

This chapter has demonstrated (a) that cost problems in the delivery of mental health services are largely associated with the costs of inpatient, not of outpatient, care; (b) that the efficacy of inpatient treatment compared with outpatient alternatives is largely unproved and therefore closer to an experimental than a well-validated treatment; (c) that the costs of mental health care are largely attributable to a relatively small number of consumers of mental health services; and (d) that mental health benefits are largely designed in an inappropriate manner.

The data presented in the chapter, along with others, suggest that mental health cost-containment efforts may best be directed to a rather small fraction of covered individuals. The data further illustrate, however, that individuals who are treated in 1 year at high cost to the indemnity plan are suggested to be at risk for further treatment in later years; thus, careful management of expenditures for such high-risk individuals may be needed. They also suggest the necessity of tracking treatment outcome over a several-year period when determining the effectiveness of employer-initiated mental health programs.

A variety of options for cost containment exist. The literature is currently mute on the differential effects of these alternatives, but employers and insurance companies do not always have the option of waiting until careful studies can be done. Present literature is sufficiently convincing, however, to suggest that benefits can be revised to encourage cost-effective behavior and that inpatient costs should be the target of special scrutiny and efforts at control.

References

Amini, F., Zilberg, N. J., Burke, E. L., & Salasnek, S. (1982). A controlled study of inpatient vs. outpatient treatment of delinquent drug abusing adolescents: One year results. *Comprehensive Psychiatry, 23,* 436–444.

Blotcky, M. J., Dimperio, T. L., & Gossett, J. T. (1984). Follow up of children treated in psychiatric hospitals: A review of studies. *American Journal of Psychiatry, 141,* 1499–1507.

Braun, P. B., Kochansky, G., Shapiro, R., Greenberg, S., Gudeman, J. E., Johnson, S., & Shore, M. F. (1981). Overview: Deinstitutionalization of psychiatric patients: A critical review of outcome studies. *American Journal of Psychiatry, 138,* 736–749.

Endicott, J., Cohen, T., Nee, J., Fleiss, J. L., & Herz, M. I. (1979). Brief vs. standard hospitalization: For whom?. *Archives of General Psychiatry, 36,* 706–712.

Glick, I. D., Hargreaves, W. A., & Goldfield, M. D. (1974). Short vs. long hospitalization: A prospective controlled study. I. The preliminary results of one-year follow up of schizophrenics. *Archives of General Psychiatry, 30,* 363–369.

Goldstein, J. M., & Horgan, C. M. (1988). Inpatient and outpatient psychiatric services: Substitutes or complements? *Hospital and Community Psychiatry, 39,* 632–637.

Gordon, T., & Breakey, W. B. (1983). A comparison of the outcomes of short- and standard-stay patients at one year follow up. *Hospital and Community Psychiatry, 34*(11), 1054–1056.

Herz, M. I., Endicott, J., & Gibbon, M. (1979). Brief hospitalization: Two-year follow-up. *Archives of General Psychiatry, 36,* 701–705.

Herz, M. I., Endicott, J., & Spitzer, R. L. (1975). Brief hospitalization of patients with families: Initial results. *American Journal of Psychiatry, 132*(4), 413–418.

Hayashida, M., Alterman, A., McLellan, T., O'Brien, C., Purtill, J., Volpicelli, J., Raphaelson, A., & Hall, C. (1989). Comparative effectiveness and costs of inpatient and outpatient detoxification of patients with mild-to-moderate alcohol withdrawal syndrome. *New England Journal of Medicine, 320,* 358–365.

Kiesler, C. A. (1982). Public and professional myths about mental hospitalization: An empirical reassessment of policy-related beliefs. *American Psychologist, 37,* 1323–1339.

Kirshner, L. A. (1982). Length of stay of psychiatric patients: A critical review and discussion. *Journal of Nervous and Mental Diseases, 170,* 27–33.

Knitzer, J. (1982). *Unclaimed children: The failure of public responsibility to children and adolescents in need of mental health services.* Washington, DC: Children's Defense Fund.

Langsley, D. G., Flomenhaft, K., & Machotka, P. (1969). Follow up evaluation of family crisis therapy. *American Journal of Orthopsychiatry, 39,* 753–759.

Langsley, D. G., & Kaplan, D. M. (1969). *The treatment of families in crisis.* New York: Grune & Stratton.

Langsley, D. G., Pittman, F., Machotka, P., & Flomenhaft, K. (1968). Family crisis therapy— results and implications. *Family Process, 7,* 145–158.

Lowman, R. L. (1987, August). *Economic incentives in the delivery of alternative mental health services.* Paper presented at the 95th Annual Convention of the American Psychological Association, New York.

Mattes, J. A., Rosen, B., & Klein, D. F. (1977). Comparison of the clinical effectiveness of "short" versus "long" stay psychiatric hospitalization: II. Results of a three-year post-hospital follow up. *Journal of Nervous and Mental Disease, 165,* 387–394.

Melton, G. B. (in press). Service models in child and adolescent mental health: What works for whom? In G. B. Melton & D. S. Hargrove (Eds.), *Planning mental health services for children and youth*. New York: Guilford.

Milasso-Sayre, L. J., Benson, P. R., Rosestein, M. J., & Manderscheid, R. W. (1986). *Use of inpatient psychiatric services by children and youth under age 18, United States, 1980* (Mental Health Statistical Note No. 175). Washington, DC: National Institute of Mental Health, Division of Biometry and Applied Sciences.

Mosher, L. R. (1983). Alternatives to psychiatric hospitalization: Why has research failed to be translated into practice? *New England Journal of Medicine, 309,* 1579–1580.

Mosher, L. R., & Menn, A. Z. (1978). Community residential treatment for schizophrenia: Two-year outcome. *Hospital and Community Psychiatry, 29,* 715–723.

Parloff, M. B. (1982). Psychotherapy research evidence and reimbursement decisions. *American Journal of Psychiatry, 139*(6), 718–727.

Parker, S., & Knoll, J. L. III (1990). Partial hospitalization: An update. *American Journal of Psychiatry, 147,* 156–160.

Pasamanick, B., Scarpitti, F. R., & Dinitz, S. (1967). *Schizophrenics in the community: An experimental study in the prevention of hospitalization.* New York: Appleton-Century-Crofts.

Rosenstock, H. A. (1985). The first 900: A nine-year longitudinal analysis of consecutive adolescent inpatients. *Adolescence, 20,* 959–973.

Weisman, G., Feinstein, A., & Thomas, C. (1969). Three-day hospitalization: A model for intensive intervention. *Archives of General Psychiatry, 21,* 620–629.

Weithorn, L. A. (1988). Mental hospitalization of troublesome youth: An analysis of skyrocketing admission rates. *Stanford Law Review, 40,* 773–838.

7

Managed Outpatient Mental Health Plans: Clinical, Ethical, and Practical Guidelines for Participation

Leonard J. Haas
and Nicholas A. Cummings

The continued emphasis on cost containment in health care, and in mental health care in particular, has stirred strong feelings (both pro and con) among psychologists in recent years. With regard to outpatient psychological treatment, it is increasingly the case that "psychotherapy" is coming to be synonymous with "brief or time-limited psychotherapy." For individual providers who examine "managed" mental health outpatient care options carefully, three questions arise forcefully: (a) Does managed mental health care present some unique set of problems for providers or patients? (b) How can psychologists make sensible decisions about participation in the "new" mental health care plans? and (c) For psychologists who are providers in managed-care environments, are there ethical or clinical considerations in deciding who should or should not be provided treatment?

The purpose of this chapter is to begin to address these questions. Although there is still much that we do not know, and there would be controversy regardless of how much data were collected, we are bold or foolish enough to attempt some provisional answers. To wit, we suggest that (a) the dilemmas presented by managed mental health care systems are not unique but are present (albeit in a less stark form) in other financing arrangements; (b) there are particular questions psychologists should ask before associating themselves with particular plans, especially about types of limitations and possible effects on the patient–provider relationship; and (c) if the therapist has appropriate training, there are very few types of patients who could not be provided with at least some benefits in a managed-care environment. We first consider the emerging context of managed care and then discuss each of these questions in somewhat more detail below. In addition, we broaden the focus on selection, to consider this question: Are there clinicians who should or should not be involved in managed mental health care plans?

Reprinted from *Professional Psychology: Research and Practice, 22*, 45–51. (1991). Copyright 1991 by the American Psychological Association.

The New Era

Increasingly in mental health service delivery, fee-for-service arrangements are a relic of the past (Cummings, 1986). The "revolution in health care" has almost guaranteed that some form of managed care will be the service used in this country by all but the extremely affluent (Zimet, 1989) or the extremely poor. Although managed care can take several forms,[1] its common ingredient is restriction on freedom (Morriem, 1988) or intrusion into the formerly private contractual world of provider and consumer. From the provider's perspective, managed mental health care plans constrain the ability of the provider to establish whatever treatment plans he or she believes will be effective for the presenting problem. From the perspective of the patient, managed care imposes some restrictions on the patient's freedom to obtain third-party reimbursement for whatever he or she thinks should be treated. And from the perspective of the offeror of insurance plans, managed mental health care offers the hope that health care costs can be contained (and the continued existence of the insurance plan promoted).

Despite many arguments and substantial evidence to the contrary (e.g., Cummings & Follette, 1976; McCall & Rice, 1983; Mumford, Schlesinger, Glass, Patrick, & Cuerdon, 1984; Schlesinger, Mumford, Glass, Patrick, & Sharfstein, 1983; VandenBos, 1983), there are still insurers who insist that increases in benefits result in increases in claims (VandenBos, 1983). Insurers also claim that reductions in benefits (often accomplished by increasing policyholders' costs for particular services) decrease service utilization. McGuire (1981) has presented perhaps the most convincing data supporting this notion of "elasticity of demand" with regard to mental health coverage. Thus, for the administrator of a managed mental health care plan, the idea of service limitation may be extremely attractive.

The Response of Psychologist Providers

Strong emotions are generated on both sides of the issue when psychologists consider the rise in managed mental health care plans. Interestingly, the focus is almost entirely on the issue of limitations to outpatient treatment, or the institution of some sort of benefit cap that might tend to shorten the length of psychotherapy. Thus, the debate seems primarily to center on time-limited[2] or brief psychotherapy versus long-term treatment. Reaction in the professional literature ranges from suggestions that psychologists have made a mis-

---

[1]Although this chapter uses the term *managed care*, it should be recognized that the term is a bit too widely used and covers several separate categories of financing arrangements. Actually, designed benefits, independent practice associations, preferred provider organizations, and health maintenance organizations are also forms of management, with greater or lesser intrusiveness into the procedures of treatment.

[2]Although we use the terms *time-limited, brief treatment,* and *short-term* therapy interchangeably, we hope it is recognized that these terms are not synonymous. Budman and Gurman (1988) suggested the term *time-sensitive* for their approach, and given our aversion to specific session limits, this is our term of choice.

take in opting to be considered health care providers to suggestions that those who fail to embrace the new systems are "dinosaurs." Even the old "symptom substitution" argument, not much in evidence since the heyday of the psychodynamic–behavioral wars, is periodically heard (e.g., time-limited treatment cannot really treat the underlying problem, but will inevitably lead to a recurrence of symptoms).

The Changing Face of Psychotherapy Economics

These questions have to some extent stemmed from perceived threats to livelihood (Cummings, 1988), but there is undeniably some ethical and clinical substance at their core. Psychologists are primarily in the business of offering outpatient mental health services, and almost all consumers of such services except for the very poor and the very wealthy depend in part on some third party to help them to afford the services. Increasingly, those third parties are imposing limits on outpatient psychotherapy to attempt to contain costs. Initially, these efforts took the form of "benefit design," or alterations in the amount of money patients must pay as they receive longer treatment (e.g., the first 5 visits at no copayment, the next 10 visits at 20% copayment, and the next 20 visits at 50% copayment). More recently, these efforts have taken the form of "management" of treatment, which inserts the third-party payor into a more active role in the treatment planning or monitoring. And, among some plans (notably, but not exclusively, certain health maintenance organizations [HMOs]), there is the feature of treatment limitation, which caps the number of sessions, not simply the number of dollars, that will be reimbursed. Although we will argue against the notion of treatment limitation by third parties, we are enthusiastic about the practitioner's use of brief methods. The ideal environment in which to contain costs would be one in which providers well trained in the rapid treatment of disorder were free to use their professional discretion in the service of their patients' welfare.

Managed Mental Health Care: Unique Threat?

Although managed-care programs in general health care were developed as a means to limit the constantly increasing cost of health care in the United States, cost containment has proved to be an elusive goal (Doleuc & Dougherty, 1985; Frank & McGuire, 1986). Rather, health care costs have escalated at a dizzying rate, and with them, mental health care costs as well. This chapter focuses primarily on outpatient mental health care plans; ironically, however, the vast proportion of mental health care costs are incurred through the use of inpatient services (Lowman, 1987; Manning, Wells, Duan, Newhouse, & Ware, 1984). Although this is a "perverse incentive" (Lowman, 1987) in that such a policy encourages the use of higher cost alternatives, the use by managed mental health care programs of limitations on outpatient benefits has continued as a cost-containment strategy. One or more of the following limitations is usually used in attempts to contain costs: increasing the patient's share of treatment costs (raising copayments); limiting dollars available per insured per year (total-cost cap); limiting treatment to conditions falling into certain diagnostic categories (prospective payment schemes); limiting treatment by number of episodes, or in inpatient settings, length of stay (treatment-episode limits); limiting treatment to specific approved techniques; and limiting treatment through requiring prior approval by "gatekeepers" (preauthorization).

Although the new realities of managed mental health care do affect the traditional relationship between provider and patient (as we discuss later), they also fail to end the risk to the survival of the plan itself, as industry spokespeople note (e.g., Jones, in VandenBos, 1983). Insurers are in constant competition for the contracts of large employers. To the extent that insurers cannot contain costs, they will suffer the consequences of loss of business to lower cost competitors or to large employers' willingness to self-insure, often with much-reduced benefit options. Hence, it is good policy for the manager of an insurance program or mental health care program to attempt to constrain costs as vigorously as possible, while of course maintaining the quality of service.

There are various means to limit the access of prospective insurance policyholders or patients to a plan or to a service. These means may be examined from clinical, fiscal, and ethical perspectives, because these are the usual types of concerns expressed about such policy decisions. That is, the clinician is most concerned about the clinical aspects of delivering quality care. The plan administrator has the clearest concern for the financial realities, because they directly affect whether the plan may survive. And both "stakeholders" (Haas & Malouf, 1989) should be concerned about the ethical dimension of their policy, in part to make it consistent with psychologists' ethical principles and in part to make it morally sound on more general grounds. A description of the options and relevant ethical concerns follows.

1. A plan may simply impose limitations on treatment. These limitations are for the present purposes being called *time limits*, although they are most clearly so primarily in HMOs. In other plans, time limits are translated into dollar limits. Thus, a plan could offer (as many do) a $2,000 yearly maximum for outpatient mental health coverage, occurring in a maximum of 50 sessions. In many HMOs, the limit is 20 sessions annually, with annual and lifetime cost caps. From a clinical perspective, this policy may be risky: Patients may be denied needed care that extends beyond their benefits. From a fiscal perspective, this policy is sensible: There is a known cap on the amount of financial risk the program takes (although there is the fiscal risk that patients may, justly or unjustly, accuse the program of depriving them of needed care). From an ethical perspective, the policy is problematic: It shifts the risk to the therapist, because therapists are ethically bound to care for their patients and not abandon them. Thus, to provide care to patients whose benefits have been exceeded puts the therapist in the position of needing to make a referral of the patient if continued treatment is appropriate. Alternatively, therapists could provide pro bono service, although doing this frequently might eventually lower the therapist's income to an unacceptable level.

— or cherry picking

2. A plan may institute no time limits but may carefully select its policyholders so that they are unlikely to exceed some (actuarially derived) time limits or expenditure limits. This is called *skimming* (McGuire, 1989), or selecting to insure those individuals who are least likely to make a claim. Although no managed-care program would admit to selecting patients in this manner, careful marketing (Nelson, Clark, Goldman, & Schore, 1989) may accomplish the same end. For example, plans may only be open to retired persons, teachers, or military dependents. However, despite the fears of critics (e.g., Nelson et al., 1989), in practice it is almost impossible to select low-utilization policyholders. One strategy that may work involves adverse selection: Lowering premiums and benefits carefully will attract those who perceive themselves to have low need for the service and to have low risk for the noncovered condition and thus expect not to need the benefits and wish to save the money. However, even if the plan administrator is judicious, this may be a relatively risky strategy in terms of financial exposure. Clinically, if it can actually be implemented, it is a relatively low-risk strategy, because it tends to amount to offering treatment to those who do not need it. Ethically, the primary problem involves informed consent; as long as the program gives policyholders clear information on the limits of coverage and they are free to choose other plans, there is no coercion into inappropriate service. However, there is the more abstract ethical concern that by selecting only low-utilization patients, the plan unfairly burdens other health insurers with higher utilization patients.

3. A plan may opt for the policy of limiting access to treatment, and limiting access to the policy itself through selection criteria or marketing strategies. There is little data on this option; however, it is likely to be fiscally the safest; a clearly known financial risk is involved. It is, on the other hand, clinically risky: Unless very clear diagnostic criteria are specified, the situation is similar to that in Paragraph 2, just discussed; it poses the danger that a patient who needs treatment will be denied it. Such a plan is potentially ethically problematic in the same way as other treatment limits are, because it changes the therapist's role to one of resource rationer and restricts his or her ability to act in the best interests of the patient.

4. A program may impose no limitations on outpatient treatment and may offer reimbursement (minus the copayment) to any policyholder. Although this is not a widespread policy (Cummings, 1988), it has proven viable when carefully implemented. Presumably, most plans avoid such an arrangement out of fear that it expands their risks uncontrollably. This policy option is clinically safe (patients who need more extensive treatment will get it); it is economically risky (the plan has no way of limiting the amount of expenses it is exposed to); and it is ethically sound (the competent and ethical provider decides in conjunction with the patient what treatment is indicated).

Overall, then, "managed" or "designed" benefits packages are not so unique; all of the issues of limiting access to treatment are present (perhaps in a less stark form) in any third-party-reimbursed scheme. All involve, in one way or another, intrusions into the traditional relationship between provider and patient. These issues will be considered next.

Considerations Before Joining a Managed-Care System

First and foremost, the prospective provider in a managed-care plan must know exactly what the plan involves and what constraints it will impose. Beyond this, several features of mental health care plans should raise questions.

1. *Who takes the risks?* In the usual arrangement, the insurer takes the risks: The plan and its benefits assume a probability of particular treatment needs, and if the patient should need more treatment, the plan reimburses for it. In managed-care plans, some of this risk is shifted to the patient: If costs go above a certain level, the patient pays. In other plans, notably HMOs, some of the risk is shifted onto providers: If costs go above the limits, or if referrals to specialists become necessary, the provider's reimbursement drops. One side effect of the shifting of risk to providers is that this tempts them to hoard resources (Morriem, 1988), in the sense that they may be reluctant to refer or extend treatment if it costs them too much.

2. *How much does the plan intrude into the patient–provider relationship?* The professional who agrees to participate in a mental health care plan incurs obligations both to the plan provider and to the patient. In the traditional doctor–patient relationship, there is substantial contractual freedom. The prototypical consumer experiences a need for a service, chooses a provider from among some alternatives, and has some degree of participation in the treatment planning process (e.g., selection of procedures if alternatives are available, agreement to follow the doctor's orders if called on to do so, and informing the provider if the treatment appears to be working). For the prototypical provider, the relationship involves loyalty to the patient; that is, the provider has the freedom to accept or decline to treat the patient, to select appropriate treatment or treatments from among those in which he or she is competent, and then to honor his or her duty to treat the patient until the presenting problem is resolved, a referral is made, or the patient discontinues treatment. In theoretical terms, the principles of beneficence, autonomy, and justice are relevant (Beauchamp & Childress, 1988). In more conventional language, the relationship is marked by freedom and responsibility: freedom to treat as the provider sees fit, and responsibility, primarily to the patient, to resolve the presenting problem. Although some commentators have argued that this arrangement provides incentives to offer more care than necessary, others (e.g., Nelson et al., 1989) have argued that it also highlights the primary loyalty of provider to consumer. The risk to the clinician participating in managed-care arrangements becomes that of balancing loyalty to the patient with responsibilities as an agent of the mental health program. If the program takes on undue risks from a particular case (e.g., the patient's care becomes too costly), the program may suffer damage, as may the therapist and other potential patients of the program.

3. *What provisions exist for exceptions to the rules?* A provider who is willing to incur the financial risk (or who works in a noncapitated arrangement) may want to continue providing treatment to a particular patient who has exceeded benefits. The provider may be tempted to change the diagnosis or the description of treatment so that the patient can be reimbursed. These

maneuvers are possible in any third-party paid arrangement, of course. However, they illustrate that tightening limits on benefits may simply challenge the creativity of clinicians loyal to their patients and that the risks of altering that loyalty extend beyond simply the escalation of costs.

4. *Are there referral resources if patient needs should exceed plan benefits?* Psychologists, like other mental health professionals, have a duty to treat the patient until the presenting problem is resolved, a referral is made, or the patient discontinues treatment. To do otherwise is to abandon the patient, and this is unethical (American Psychological Association [APA], 1990). Thus, a key question before joining a plan that limits benefits may well become, How do practitioners avoid abandoning their patients without going bankrupt?

5. *Does the plan provide assistance or training in helping the provider to achieve treatment goals?* An alternative to the dilemma just mentioned involves the clinician in becoming more knowledgeable about short-term treatment options. A variety of brief therapy approaches exists (Budman, 1978; Sperry, 1989). If prospective providers have not been trained in these approaches, plans either should not select them or should make provisions to train them appropriately.

6. *Does the plan minimize economic incentives to hospitalize patients?* The "perverse incentives" noted earlier operate in many plans. Providers should carefully investigate their existence and perhaps lobby for alternative incentive systems.

7. *Are there ways in which the plan is open to provider input?* Given the proliferation of benefit options and plan arrangements, it is essential that some feedback mechanisms be built into these plans. Otherwise, the provider becomes simply an employee rather than a professional treating patients.

8. *Do plans clearly inform their policyholders of the limits of benefits?* Just as providers have loyalties to both other parties in the system, they should avoid being trapped in the middle, having to explain benefit limits to naive patients after the benefit limits have been reached.

Of course, the ideal policy for a managed mental health care program is one that does not create dual loyalties among therapists and that provides benefits both to specific patients in need of services and to potential patients who may require program resources in the future. This is a difficult policy option to implement because pressing, immediate needs are those most likely to claim our loyalties even though alleviating present needs may increase the suffering of patients who will have needs in the future.

Selection of Appropriate Patients

Once psychologists have decided to become providers in managed-care plans, additional choices present themselves. An issue that has generated much debate (but unfortunately, few data) is the question of whether there are certain prospective patients who should be excluded from "managed" (e.g., time-limited) treatment, or patients for whom it is indicated, or both. If a plan limits treatment, it is both clinically and ethically problematic to offer services to inappropriate cases (e.g., those who would deteriorate under the proposed treatment limits). However, there is much debate about which cases are inappropriate. Because there are few or no reliable data to suggest who might deteriorate, perhaps a way to reduce some of these risks is to offer a pretherapy trial of one to three sessions (as Budman & Gurman, 1988, suggested) to determine the patient's response to brief, focused therapy.

Exclusion Criteria

MacKenzie (1989), in a review of recent developments in brief psychotherapy, suggested that there is reasonable agreement in the literature regarding the exclusion of certain types of patients from brief psychotherapy. Unfortunately, these appear not to be differential criteria (i.e., they would be important exclusion criteria from any sort of verbal treatment, short or long term). Specifically, MacKenzie listed three criteria: patients unable to attend to the process of verbal interaction; patients with diagnoses for which other treatment modalities take precedence; and patients with a characterological style that "precludes the likelihood of enduring through the psychological work" (p. 745). The first category of patients includes those suffering from retardation, delirium, dementia, and active psychosis; the second category includes patients with acute panic disorder, major affective disorders, and schizophreniform disorders; and the third category includes those with "a history of repeated serious suicide attempts, entrenched alcohol or substance abuse, or chronic obsessional or phobic patterns" (p. 745). Mackenzie did note that there is some disagreement regarding whether brief therapy is clearly contraindicated for all of these conditions. For example, Davanloo (1980) advocated brief approaches specifically for obsessional and phobic symptoms. Horowitz et al. (1984) additionally recommended brief therapy for patients with histrionic, compulsive, borderline, and narcissistic character disorders, although with limited goals. Budman and Gurman (1988) and Koss and Butcher (1986) made similar points about using time-sensitive therapy to treat, respectively, personality disorders or Axis II disorders listed in the third edition of the *Diagnostic and Statistical Manual of Mental Disorders,* (American Psychiatric Association, 1980). Burlingame, Fuhriman, Paul, and Ogles (1989) summarized criteria for involvement in short-term therapy as follows: The patient should have focal concerns; the concerns should be clear cut and have emerged at identifiable points in time; there should be a history of at least one significant attachment; there should not be a presenting picture of chronic anger, psychopathy, organicity, or psychosis; and the patient should be in subjective psychological distress. Clearly, excluding patients on these criteria from inclusion in managed mental health care programs is impossible. More typically, selection is made by limiting the eligibility for service to particular diagnostic categories (e.g., the plan does not cover situational adjustment disorders, or the plan does not cover personality disorders).

Within plans that reimburse only for the treatment of certain diagnostic categories, the frequently encountered limitation on the allowed number of sessions must be considered. Those who claim that such caps are appropriate argue that time limits focus the time and efforts of the clinician in a way that makes the treatment more cost-effective. Those who argue against this notion (e.g., Cummings & VandenBos, 1979) argue that a carefully trained clinician can quickly target symptoms and treat them without imposing time limits on patients and incurring all the "loyalty risks" noted earlier. Further, Budman and Gurman (1988) have shown that repeated "doses" of brief therapy can have the same effect as, or perhaps even a better effect than one, dose of treatment. Budman and Gurman also present compelling theoretical arguments that brief, time-sensitive treatment can offer benefits that may in some cases be superior to time-unlimited therapy. Data also exist (Smith, Glass, & Miller, 1980) that treatment response is not dependent on treatment duration. Thus, the evidence suggests that brief treatment should not be denied, and in fact may be effectively provided, to patients with a variety of diagnostic conditions previously thought inappropriate.

Inclusion Criteria

MacKenzie (1989, p. 746), suggests that "once exclusion criteria have been applied, the remaining patients can then be assessed on criteria that make them suitable for inclusion." He notes that the literature points to the following criteria for successful treatment: capacity to relate, psychological-mindedness, motivation, response to "trial interpretation," and adaptational strengths. These criteria, like exclusionary ones, are quite similar to those that predict good response to any form of psychotherapy.

An additional, ethical method for determining whether or not time-limited treatment is indicated is to consider the alternatives: Would the patient really be worse off with no treatment than with only a few sessions?

Effects on Therapist–Patient Relationship

It is also useful for the clinician to consider the likely treatment relationship that will develop with particular kinds of patients, especially with respect to the forces on the relationship that participation in a managed-care plan will emphasize. These issues revolve around the specific match of patient and therapist and raise the question of whether some patients provoke efforts in certain therapists to collude with them to "beat the system." Conversely, some patients may so alienate certain therapists with their sense of entitlement or their dependency that they evoke tendencies to prematurely eject them from the system even when the benefits might be available. Clearly, these tendencies are possible in treatment covered by traditional insurance plans, but the symbolic presence of the "manager" or third party intensifies the issues in vulnerable therapist–patient pairs.

An additional issue, especially in long-term or chronic conditions, is the temptation to "dump" the patient on public mental health facilities when his or her benefits have been exhausted. Again, these temptations are not unique to managed-care systems, but the risk that a third party (e.g., the HMO administrator) may exert pressure on the provider is still present.

An additional risk that should be addressed is related to the little-used option noted here earlier to provide additional pro bono service. In some therapist–patient dyads this can take the form of the therapist sacrificing him- or herself for the benefit of the patient, providing additional (unreimbursed) sessions, going beyond session limits or time limits with the patient, and so forth. Such therapists, who break the rules or in some way circumvent them to continue providing services to those in the plan who have used up their share of the resources, may be "poaching," in the terms of Morreim (1988), because the resources (time, energy, etc.) that they use for the "favored" patients are less available for other patients' use.

Selection of Clinicians

In effect, the implication of these findings is that selection of therapists (and appropriate training of therapists, as Burlingame et al., 1989, suggest) is more important than selection of patients for time-limited treatment. The ability of the therapist to focus on achievable, specific treatment goals, and to be active and more directive in conducting the treatment, cannot be taken for granted. Family-therapy researchers have suggested that therapists can be arrayed on a dimension of passivity–activity and that effective family therapists are highly active and directive. Additional research into therapist characteristics in individual treatment (e.g., Lambert, 1986) also suggests that therapist activity level is important in determining outcome. These suggestions are at present only implied by the literature. Much more research is needed regarding the nature of the interaction between therapist training, experience, activity level, and type of presenting problem in determining outcome. One likely implication of these lines of inquiry is that therapists who are not comfortable with a more active, directive role should probably avoid involvement in managed mental health care programs.

In addition, it is becoming clear that brief therapy modalities are not simply the abbreviated forms of long-term therapy approaches to which most clinicians were exposed in graduate school (Sperry, 1989). A small but growing literature (e.g., Budman, 1978) describes various approaches to time-limited therapy. Thus, it is likely to soon be the case that brief therapy will encompass its own set of skills. Therapists who are not competent in brief therapy or therapies should also probably avoid involvement in managed mental health care programs.

Finally, the foregoing discussion has briefly described the type of intrusion in the traditional doctor–patient relationship likely to occur in managed mental-health care programs. Therapists who strongly resent such intrusions also should probably avoid involvement in managed mental health care programs. Perhaps a corollary of this is that therapists who cannot endorse the structure of the plan they are involved in should also look elsewhere, or perhaps, consistent with Principle 3 of the "Ethical Principles of Psychologists" (APA,

1990), attempt to change the arrangements. To act otherwise is to risk colluding with the patient and "acting out" against the plan.

Additional Ethical Issues

Consideration of additional ethical issues in managed mental health care plans brings several to the forefront. First, as noted earlier, the issue of competence is crucial. Consistent with the ethical obligation to offer services within the domain of their competence, psychologists must be capable of delivering service in a time-limited context if they are to be involved in managed-care plans.

Second is the issue of informed consent. The prospective patient must be given clear information about the benefits to which he or she is entitled and clear information about the limits of treatment as the clinician envisions them.

A third issue of ethical importance concerns divided loyalties. Third-party payment arrangements always elicit such issues, but never so clearly as in managed mental health care plans. The principal of fidelity (Beauchamp & Childress, 1988) demands that the provider or professional be loyal to those with whom he or she has a contractual relationship. Thus, if a therapist agrees to work in a managed health-care program, he or she should believe in the service philosophy it endorses. If the therapist agrees to work with a particular patient, he or she should be loyal to that patient's interests. (This is part of what is meant by a fiduciary relationship.) The "Ethical Principles of Psychologists" (APA, 1990) focuses on fidelity in Principle 6, in terms of the psychologist's obligation to obtain informed consent from consumers, and on avoiding relationships in which there is a conflict of interest that may impair his or her objectivity. On this last point, the "Ethical Principles of Psychologists" (APA, 1990) is also clear: When demands of an organization conflict with the ethics code, psychologists attempt to bring the conflict to the attention of relevant parties and resolve it. In this case, the conflict would likely be between the demands of the plan that reimbursement for treatment cease or change versus the needs of the patient and the psychologist's ethical responsibility to act for the benefit of the client ("welfare of the consumer"). Psychologists may have a corollary obligation to ensure that plans with which they are associated have mechanisms to receive their input and recommendations for change.

Discussion and Conclusion

Although the emergence of various innovations (some would call them "throwbacks") in financing mental health care has generated much debate, there are few widely accepted empirical findings on which to base decisions about participation and patient selection. What can clearly be established is this: The forces unleashed by the managed mental health care revolution are different in degree but not in kind from those already pressing on patients and their therapists in existing third-party reimbursement schemes. Providers can and should attempt to educate plan administrators about cost-effective alternatives. In addition, providers should attempt to educate patients or plan purchasers (usually large employers) regarding the nature of the benefits they are being offered. In a sense, patients who are willing to pay higher fees for treatment on an outpatient basis are actually subsidizing those patients who wait until they are in need of (or their providers believe they are in need of) more costly inpatient treatment.

The practical implications of these changes are (a) time-sensitive treatment must be considered the initial approach, although its specifics may vary, depending on the therapist's theoretical leanings and the condition of the patient; (b) financing plans vary in their capacity for flexibility and their openness to provider input, and psychologists should be cautious about which plans they join; (c) the evidence for negative effects of time-sensitive treatment on various severe and chronic disorders is equivocal, and the primary concern should be "do no harm" (MacKenzie, 1989); (d) there is encouraging evidence concerning repeated brief "doses" of treatment, with clearly articulated and limited goals, for chronic and severe conditions (Budman & Gurman, 1988); and (e) psychologists should continually be aware of the loyalty conflicts to which they will be exposed and prepare themselves to confront these dilemmas forthrightly. An implication that this chapter does not permit us to expand on is that psychologists need support systems to help them navigate these environments and should work to foster open discussions of these problems with informed colleagues.

Clearly, the battle to contain costs should not be fought in the outpatient mental health clinics; the major fiscal drains on the system are elsewhere. But equally clearly, psychologists will gain little by doing nothing more than complaining about this fact. Carefully selecting one's training, carefully selecting the plans one associates with, and carefully selecting the interventions one attempts with clients are likely to be the keys to satisfactory professional life in the "new era."

References

American Psychiatric Association. (1980). *Diagnostic and statistical manual of mental disorders* (3rd ed.). Washington, DC: Author.

American Psychological Association. (1990). Ethical principles of psychologists (amended June 2, 1989). *American Psychologist, 45,* 390–395.

Beauchamp, T., & Childress, W. (1988). *Principles of biomedical ethics* (3rd ed.). Baltimore: Johns Hopkins University Press.

Budman, S. H. (1978). *Forms of brief therapy.* New York: Guilford Press.

Budman, S. H., & Gurman, A. S. (1988). *Theory and practice of brief therapy.* New York: Guilford Press.

Burlingame, G. M., Fuhriman, A., Paul, S., & Ogles, B. (1989). Implementing a time-limited therapy program: Differential effects of training and experience. *Psychotherapy, 26,* 303–313.

Cummings, N. A. (1986). The dismantling of our health system: Strategies for the survival of psychological practice. *American Psychologist, 41,* 426–431.

Cummings, N. A. (1988). Emergence of the mental health complex: Adaptive and maladaptive responses. *Professional Psychology: Research and Practice, 19,* 308–315.

Cummings, N. A., & Follette, W. T. (1976). Brief psychotherapy and medical utilization: An eight year follow-up. In H. Dorken & Associates (Eds.), *The professional psychologist today: New developments in law, health insurance, and health practice.* San Francisco: Jossey-Bass.

Cummings, N. A., & VandenBos, G. R. (1979). The general practice of psychology. *Professional Psychology: Research and Practice, 10,* 430–440.

Davanloo, H. (1980). (Ed.). *Short-term dynamic psychotherapy.* New York: Aronson.

Doleuc, D. A., & Dougherty, L. J. (1985). The counterrevolution in financing health care. *Hastings Center Report, 15,* 19–29.

Frank, R., & McGuire, T. (1986). A review of studies of the impact of insurance on the demand and utilization of specialty mental health services. *Health Services Research, 21,* 241–266.

Haas, L. J., & Malouf, J. L. (1989). *Keeping up the good work: A practitioner's guide to mental health ethics.* Sarasota, FL: Professional Resource Exchange.

Horowitz, M., Marmar, C., Krupnick, J., Wilner, N., Kaltreider, N., & Wallerstein, R. (1984). *Personality styles and brief psychotherapy.* New York: Guilford Press.

Koss, M., & Butcher, J. (1986). Research on brief psychotherapy. In S. Garfield & A. Bergin (Eds.), *Handbook of psychotherapy and behavior change* (3rd ed.). New York: Wiley.

Lambert, M. (1986). Research on therapist characteristics as they impact therapeutic outcome. In S. Garfield & A. Bergin (Eds.), *Handbook of psychotherapy and behavior change* (3rd ed.). New York: Wiley.

Lowman, R. L. (1987, August). *Economic incentives in the delivery of alternative mental health services.* Paper presented at the 95th Annual Convention of the American Psychological Association, New York, NY.

Manning, W. G., Wells, K. B., Duan, N., Newhouse, J. P., & Ware, J. E. (1984). Cost sharing and the use of ambulatory mental health services. *American Psychologist, 39,* 1077–1084.

MacKenzie, K. R. (1989). Recent developments in brief psychotherapy. *Hospital and Community Psychiatry, 39,* 742–752.

McGuire, T. (1981). *Financing psychotherapy.* Cambridge, MA: Ballinger.

McGuire, T. G. (1989). Outpatient benefits for mental health services in medicare: Alignment with the private sector? *American Psychologist, 44,* 818–824.

McCall, N., & Rice, T. (1983). A summary of the Colorado clinical psychology/expanded mental health benefits experiment. *American Psychologist, 38,* 1279–1291.

Morreim, E. H. (1988). Cost containment: Challenging fidelity and justice. *Hastings Center Report, 18,* 20–25.

Mumford, E., Schlesinger, H. J., Glass, G., Patrick, C., & Cuerdon, B. (1984). A new look at evidence about reduced medical utilization following mental health treatment. *American Journal of Psychiatry, 141,* 1145–1158.

Nelson, L. J., Clark, H. W., Goldman, R. L., & Schore, J. E. (1989). Taking the train to a world of strangers: Health care marketing and ethics. *Hastings Center Report, 19,* 36–43.

Schlesinger, H. J., Mumford, E., Glass, G. V., Patrick, C., & Sharfstein, S. (1983). Mental health treatment and medical care utilization in a fee-for-service system: Outpatient mental health treatment following the onset of a chronic disease. *American Journal of Public Health, 73,* 422–429.

Smith, M. L., Glass, G. V., & Miller, T. I. (1980). *The benefits of psychotherapy.* Baltimore: Johns Hopkins University Press.

Sperry, L. (1989). Contemporary approaches to brief psychotherapy: A comparative analysis. *Individual psychology: The journal of Adlerian therapy, research and practice, 45,* 3–25.

VandenBos, G. R. (1983). Health financing, service utilization, and national policy: A conversation with Stan Jones. *American Psychologist, 38,* 948–955.

Zimet, C. N. (1989). The mental health care revolution: Will psychology survive? *American Psychologist, 44,* 703–708.

8

Realities of Mental Health Practice in Managed-Care Settings

*Linda M. Richardson
and Carol Shaw Austad*

Although health care providers as well as consumers have responded to the rapid growth in managed health care with mixed emotions and often with resistance (Hoyt, 1985), it is clear that this form of health care delivery is here to stay. The question is no longer whether managed care will survive but rather, what form or forms will it take?

Whatever their ambivalence about or resistance to managed mental health care, psychologists in clinical practice may find it difficult to survive financially if they should choose not to participate in such systems, because the majority of the American population will likely obtain their future health care through some form of managed health care organization (Cummings, 1986; Zimet, 1989). Adaptation to today's changing health service delivery systems requires that clinicians alter their traditional attitudes toward mental health care, as well as their clinical, administrative, organizational, and financial practices.

This chapter provides information to assist psychologists in adapting to the unprecedented changes that are occurring in mental health service delivery. More specifically, the chapter addresses the following subjects: typical mental health benefits, advantages and disadvantages of managed mental health care from both the provider's and the consumer's perspectives, alternative ways in which psychologists can interact with managed-care systems, common types of financial arrangements for providers, and clinical and organizational issues in managed care.

The Benefit Package in Managed Health Care

Managed health care has been variously defined. The lack of standard definitions for the various types of managed-care arrangements (i.e., health maintenance organization [HMO], preferred provider organization [PPO], independent practice association [IPA], etc.) makes accurate comparisons difficult

Reprinted from *Professional Psychology: Research and Practice, 22*, 52–59. (1991). Copyright 1991 by the American Psychological Association.

(Walworth, O'Donnell, Pearson, & Solem, 1987). However, Anderson and Fox (1987) noted that the essence of managed health care is attention to both health care delivery and health care costs in an effort to combine cost savings and quality care.

Despite the diversity of managed health care systems, there are some typical benefit plans. In a survey of HMOs (Levin, Glasser, & Jaffee, 1988), it was found that most have some form of mental health coverage. Of those offering mental health benefits, nearly all provided some form of outpatient services, over half provided inpatient services, and two thirds offered coverage for alcohol and drug problems (although in nearly one third of these, coverage was limited to detoxification only). Typically, substance-abuse coverage was provided as an add-on rider rather than as part of the basic coverage.

To qualify for low-interest federal loans for start-up or expansion costs, federally chartered HMOs (which can include for-profit entities) must abide by the HMO federal guidelines for mental health services. The HMO Public Service Act of 1973 (Public Law 93-222) and its subsequent amendments in 1976, 1978, and 1981 (Levin, 1988; Levin et al., 1988) require that federally chartered HMOs provide the following mental health services as part of their health coverage: (a) outpatient mental health services consisting of short-term evaluation and crisis intervention, up to 20 sessions, and (b) medical care and appropriate referral services for chemical dependency. The HMO Act and its revisions did not mandate inpatient care, nor was long-term care a required component. Some nonfederally chartered HMOs may also follow these guidelines to be competitive with the federally qualified HMOs, whereas others may choose not to observe them, presumably as a cost-saving measure (Flinn, McMahon, & Collins, 1987).

In a national survey of 304 managed health care organizations, Levin et al. (1988) found that 97% of surveyed HMOs offered some type of mental health coverage in their basic benefit, 79% offered 20 sessions of outpatient care, and 67% offered some type of substance-abuse benefits. Levin et al. also found that over the 10-year period from 1976 to 1986, both mental health and drug and alcohol treatment benefits in managed health care organizations remained constant, with a median outpatient therapy benefit of 20 sessions per member per year and inpatient benefits of 30 days per member per year. Apparently, what was mandated as minimal coverage has become the maximum benefit in many settings. Furthermore, although clients often expect to receive full mental health benefits (e.g., 20 outpatient sessions) when they seek care, they may be upset to discover barriers to receiving them, such as copayments, complicated screening methodologies, and treatment limitations. Because HMOs are usually "at risk" for the use of mental health services, there is an obvious incentive to curtail service use. The ability to do so is not unlimited, of course, because clients who become dissatisfied with restricted access to services may simply drop their membership; and, if HMOs become too aggressive in denying or limiting services, there is the risk of violating the federal charter.

The theoretically mandated health benefits in HMOs do not appear unreasonable when compared with national statistics on mental health care use. Research has demonstrated that 50% of all mental health clients are improved in 8 or fewer sessions, and 75–80% in 26 or fewer sessions (Carr-Kaffashan, 1989; Goodstein, 1986; Pallak, 1987). Moreover, the modal client stays in outpatient treatment for only 1 visit, with the average length of treatment being 4 to 6 visits regardless of the type of treatment or the setting (Budman, 1989; Phillips, 1988). The mental health service attrition curve developed by Phillips (1985) shows that only 50% of all clients return for the 1st therapy session after the intake interview, and a declining number continue in therapy, so that by the 5th or 6th session 70% of all clients have left therapy, and only a very small percentage of clients remain in treatment after the 10th session. This use pattern applies to all types of clients, whether treated with short-term or long-term therapy, regardless of the theoretical approach. Similar utilization statistics are found in HMOs.

Economic factors, however, may still make HMOs or other managed-care plans seem attractive, to both consumers and employers. For example, a common indemnity (traditional group insurance) plan such as Blue Cross/Blue Shield 2000 usually covers only 50% of the costs of outpatient psychotherapy up to a limit of from $600 to $2,000 per year, depending on the particulars of the plan (Zimet, 1989). To receive psychotherapy for 20 weeks a year (the typical HMO benefit) at a conservative assumed rate of $80 per session, the client with a traditional insurance plan would have to pay out-of-pocket between $800 and $1,000 (Austad, 1988; Zimet, 1989), whereas the managed-care member would typically pay a small copayment or no copayment for 20 sessions. Levin et al.'s (1988) survey of HMOs found that HMOs charged a mean copayment of $15 per visit for outpatient mental health care, and this copayment was charged only after an average of 5 visits.

Although the mental health benefits typically found in managed-care plans have been severely criticized by some for their limited coverage, when examined closely, they do not differ greatly from the coverage offered by traditional indemnity plans. However, if the economic interests of managed-health plans result in more barriers to accessing mental health care than traditional indemnity plans (e.g., mandatory physician referrals, long waiting lists, triage screening prior to therapist assignment, approval of therapy sessions in small numbers), the plan may be less attractive.

Client payments and other aspects of traditional mental health care that have been considered important parts of the therapeutic process change character in managed health systems. When there is little or no out-of-pocket expense, a sense of personal sacrifice may not be experienced in the therapy. Yet, the importance of such sacrifice to therapeutic effectiveness has been challenged. Interestingly, mental health service use rates, contrary to expectations, do not accelerate rapidly when financial barriers to care are removed. Prepaid mental health clients appear to exhibit no higher utilization rates than fee-for-service adult consumers (Blackwell, Gutmann, & Gutmann, 1988). Similarly, clinicians have expressed concern that clients with chronic mental health needs who belong to managed care plans may be denied needed mental health services because of the federal HMO guidelines, which focus on brief, crisis-oriented care only (Talbott, 1981); in fact, it has been estimated that approximately 10% of those who seek mental health care cannot be managed within the usual HMO restrictions (Carr-Kaffashan, 1989). However, the aged, poor, and chronically ill (groups with high mental health service needs) are typically underrepresented in many managed-care or HMO systems because most such plans are directed to employed persons and their dependents (and therefore younger and healthier populations; Feldman, 1986).

Managed Health Care: Advantages and Disadvantages for Providers and Consumers

Providers

Clinicians can participate in managed health care in a variety of ways. The type of health care system, as well as the specific nature of the clinician's relationship with that system, will significantly affect all aspects of the clinician's participation. The provider may interact with various types of managed-care systems, including HMOs, IPAs, and PPOs. An HMO provides specified health services using a restricted group of providers at a fixed cost to the consumer; a PPO buys health care from specific providers usually at a discounted rate, sometimes with a small percentage of fees withheld until year's end. The incentive for providers is the promise of increased volume of clients. An IPA allows consumers to choose independent practice providers but holds back a portion of the fees from the providers, who may be reimbursed either on a fee-for-service basis or on a capitated basis (Cummings & Duhl, 1987; Flinn et al., 1987; Gurevitz, 1984); *capitation* refers to a fixed monthly or annual payment according to the number of persons covered by the managed-care plan; payment is unrelated to the amount of service provided. HMOs, and to a lesser extent, PPOs have built-in incentives to use less costly and presumably less well-trained mental health professionals.

Clinicians' financial arrangements with different types of managed-care systems vary. In a staff HMO, clinicians are salaried. Group HMOs may remunerate mental health professionals using either salaried, fee-for-service, or capitated systems. Providers in PPOs and IPAs are typically reimbursed on a fee-for-service or capitated basis.

Clinicians as Employees: Staff- and Group-Model HMOs

In the staff-model HMO, clinicians are employed full time or part time by the HMO. Group-model HMOs are operated very similarly, but some employees (generally physicians) also own an interest in the HMO. (Two well-known examples of these types of HMOs are Community Health Care Plan in New Haven, Connecticut, which is a staff-model HMO, and Kaiser Permanente in California, which is a group-model HMO.)

Advantages to the provider of being on staff in an HMO include a steady clientele, stable salary, often excellent benefits, the opportunity to practice in an interdisciplinary setting, involvement in the total health care of the client with the goals of integrating and coordinating services, a predictable work schedule, availability of colleagues, minimal involvement with fee collection, a wide range of clients and problems, the possibility of implementing programs for target persons or problems (or both), and the opportunity to use a wide variety of clinical skills. Disadvantages to this arrangement include restrictions on the amount and type of mental health care that can be provided, participation in on-call service, strong emphasis on short-term treatment for all types of problems, heavy caseloads and little time for reading or reflection, limited involvement with clients, little or no control over numbers or types of clients seen, lack of choice over clients seen, divided loyalty between client and HMO, concern over quality of care and restricted focus of treatment (typically limited to the presenting problem).

Clinicians as Contractors: PPOs and IPAs

In contractual managed-care arrangements, clinicians are not employees but rather independent agents. Although specific features may vary with differing organizational entities, the issues related to being a contractor are similar. Clients are encouraged to use the contracted providers because of their reduced fees, low or absent deductibles, and small or nonexistent copayments, whereas providers are "preferred" because they agree to reduce fees and to adhere to rules and parameters of the managed-care system or submit to utilization review, or both (De Lissovoy, Rice, Gabel, & Gelzer, 1987). Clinicians, whether solo practitioners or members of a group practice, are selectively contracted to participate, presumably on the basis of their ability to deliver cost-effective clinical services.

As a contractor, the solo practitioner or group practice may have little voice in the organization's decision making and little or no choice in selection of types of cases with which to work. Relationships with other managed health care providers may be limited. Typically, the clinician is paid a reduced fee and may assume some financial risk if paid on a capitated basis.

Clinicians, especially those in group practices, may be contracted to provide all mental health services to a managed health care organization when such services are not offered within the organization. Others may be contracted to provide care either because of an excess volume of clients within the managed-care organization or because they can offer treatment to long-term cases or those requiring certain types of specialized expertise.

The Consumer

For consumers, there are many advantages to joining a managed health care plan. Early on, these plans were especially appealing because membership costs of HMOs were typically lower than those of traditional indemnity plans. Now, however, they may be equal to or somewhat higher than for traditional health insurance. Other potential advantages for the client include ease of access to a variety of health services and limited paperwork in filing claims

(Shulman, 1989). Managed health care systems may also remove financial and other barriers to the use of specialty services such as mental health (Lange, Chandler-Guy, Forti, Foster-Moore, & Rohman, 1988). Also, because HMOs have not been permitted to exclude clients with preexisting conditions, persons who might not otherwise be insurable can obtain much-needed health coverage. Overall, prepaid systems can be very attractive, especially to younger people who may appreciate the generous outpatient benefits (Flinn et al., 1987).

However, managed health care plans also have disadvantages. Perhaps the single most troublesome limitation is that enrollees in typical HMOs must choose their health care providers from those designated by the system instead of having free choice. Moreover, most managed systems do not permit their subscribers to consult a specialist directly but instead require that a client receive a referral from the primary health care provider to the specialist. This gatekeeping system is an effort to reduce unnecessary and costly visits to specialists. If such a gatekeeping system is used in a health care organization with a small number of practitioners, other disadvantages may occur, including long waiting periods for appointments and assignment to nonpreferred providers or treatments. Especially for mental health services, few providers or areas of specialization may be available.

Accessing Mental Health Services

Clients access mental health care in managed-care systems either by booking appointments directly with mental health care providers, or more typically, by referral from their primary health care providers, usually family physicians. In the former system, they may be assessed by telephone or in person to determine their eligibility and appropriateness for care. The gatekeeping approach is intended to prevent unnecessary and thus costly care, though this system assumes that primary health care providers are qualified to assess mental health needs. Triage or screening interviews may be conducted by designated personnel, typically registered nurses, who determine whether mental health care is needed and, if so, to whom the referral will be made. Alternatively, the assessing clinician may become the therapist.

Once a case has been assigned to a clinician and therapy has begun, treatment is usually reviewed periodically by a utilization review committee. Typically, this review involves paper scrutiny, although occasionally it requires the clinician to make an oral presentation to the committee. Feedback is then provided to the clinician about the adequacy of the progress of the case. In practice, various barriers to further treatment may be imposed, such as an upper limit being placed on the number of additional treatment sessions permitted. Treatment may not be allowed to continue until this review process occurs and reauthorization of care is granted. In other instances, the clinician has a session or two automatically granted beyond the review point to allow time for the review to occur.

In other models, the number of treatment sessions is determined by the initial referral sources (either the primary-care providers or the triage personnel). Unfortunately, they may lack mental health knowledge. Reviewers and referral sources may also have incentives to curtail or severely limit services because their livelihood may be affected. Not without controversy, some managed-care systems provide financial incentives to their primary care personnel and reviewers for not referring clients to specialists.

Still other managed-care systems may penalize those providers who make too many referrals for diagnostic testing or specialty consultations. The General Accounting Office of the federal government has studied these practices and concluded that they adversely affect care (General Accounting Office, 1988). Of special concern are systems in which bonuses are paid on physician-specific performance (rather than on group performance), with a portion of health care cost savings paid as a bonus, and physician performance measured over a short period. A proposed law forbids physician bonus plans in HMOs.

Financial Arrangements

Fee for Service

In the traditional fee-for-service model, the provider bills the consumer for a specified amount, typically on the basis of the amount of time spent delivering the service. Until recently, the dollar amount for a service was provider driven. Usual and customary fees were generally accepted, sometimes with defined parameters as to how fees could be changed. Now, the provider alone no longer determines the fees because referral sources may demand that a specific fee schedule be used in exchange for their business. PPOs represent an attempt to save the fee-for-service method of payment by regulating the cost of treatment in the context of a traditional reimbursement plan.

Prospective Payment

As part of the effort to control spiraling health-care costs, Health Care Financing Administration (HCFA) payers, dissatisfied with the fee-for-service models, have developed a prospective payment system for the costs of services to Medicare clients (Hsia, Krushat, Fagan, Tebutt, & Kusserow, 1988). In this methodology, HCFA pays fixed prices for treatment of each of 468 diagnosis-related groups (DRGs) to hospitals on the basis of a client's diagnoses coded at discharge, regardless of the amount of service actually provided. Attempts are being made to establish DRGs for mental disorders as well.

Capitation

In the capitated system, a provider or a group of providers agree (within defined parameters) to deliver all of the mental health care required by a given population for a fixed cost per member or employee. In this system, providers assume financial risk for a given population because payment to the provider is the same regardless of the amount of service rendered.

Clinical Practice Issues

Today's mental health practitioners are pressured to alter their service delivery practices to meet the demands of the new health care environment. More specifically, they may be forced to be eclectic, versatile, knowledgeable about which therapeutic techniques are most appropriate with particular types of clients, and able to demonstrate the efficacy of their work. Clinicians may be forced to examine their belief systems and attitudes toward mental health care and adjust them to fit the new managed-care environment. Fundamental questions arise: Is long-term therapy superior to short-term therapy? When is inpatient care preferable to outpatient care? Should mental health care be standardized like physical health care by designing treatment protocols for each major diagnosis? and How does quality control, utilization review, and the intrusive presence of the third-party payer affect mental health care?

Long-Term Versus Short-Term Psychotherapy

For many clinicians, especially those trained in psychoanalytic or psychodynamic theory and practice, short-term treatment is often considered "second class" compared with long-term, insight-oriented therapy (Davanloo, 1979). Although surveys of psychologists' self-described theoretical orientations have typically shown that psychologists are moving away from psychodynamic models and toward more eclectic models, a significant minority still prefers the psychodynamic models. Among clinicians in HMOs, the psychodynamic orientation still prevails, according to a survey being conducted by Carol Shaw Austad. Resistance to short-term psychotherapy may be expressed in a number of ways, including the belief that more treatment is better than less treatment, that long-term therapy is better than short-term therapy, and that the probing of unconscious conflicts is superior to treating stated presenting problems (Berkman, Bassos, & Post, 1988; Hoyt, 1985). It can be threatening for clinicians to discover that shorter and less costly therapy is as effective as (or more effective than) long-term treatment in producing change. Many clinicians resent having their practices subject to external controls, thereby threatening their perceived autonomy (Zimet, 1989). More specifically, they may not like mandated short-term approaches or having their work scrutinized by utilization review committees. However, if they can be persuaded of the benefits of short-term therapy for their clients and the personal benefits of treatment reviews, their attitudes may become more positive toward these practices.

Educative approaches, including the use of research findings, may help to change attitudes. Literature demonstrating that clients do improve with short-term care is likely to alter resistant therapists' attitudes. Education can also improve short-term therapy skills (Budman, 1989). Short-term treatment is not just long-term treatment conducted in a briefer time period. Clinicians not trained in brief therapy, who yet work in managed-care settings that demand short-term, cost-effective treatment, are more likely to be dissatisfied and terminate their involvement early, their clients are more likely to be dissatisfied with their care, the treatment is more likely to be unstructured and therefore take longer and hence cost more, and the therapists are more likely to lack faith in being able to obtain positive outcomes from brief treatment and likely to communicate this pessimism to their clients (Budman, 1989).

In addition to brief treatment skills, the clinician must have expertise in rapid assessment in order to be able to identify the core psychological issues quickly and match each client with the most appropriate therapist and intervention (Berkman et al., 1988). Short-term work is typically more difficult than long-term work because its aim is to accomplish significant change in a brief period, and this requires that the therapist be more active.

When selecting brief-therapy interventions for specific clients with specific problems, several factors must be considered, including what intervention is likely to be most appropriate, least intrusive, and least costly in terms of time and money (Austad, DeStefano, & Kisch, 1988). The client's strengths and motivation for change must also be considered. Austad et al. recommend the following therapies to be particularly appropriate for use in HMO settings, whether in individual, group, or family work: crisis and problem-solving therapy, personal-growth therapy, developmental therapy, educative therapy, and chronic psychiatric problem-solving therapy. Budman (1989) has developed two types of interventions specifically for managed-care settings: (a) a developmental model focusing on the client's developmental stage as the context for the problem and (b) a crisis-intervention model. Cummings (1988) has proposed an intermittent model in which clients may seek mental health care periodically over their lifetimes in much the same way as they seek medical care from a family doctor; treatment is therefore not viewed as a once and forever intervention.

When practicing in a managed-care setting, clinicians may be called on to use a variety of treatment modalities. In addition to such cost-effective treatment modalities as group therapy (in managed care, a member typically can receive twice as many group sessions as individual sessions) and family therapy, clinicians can also avail themselves of such approaches as bibliotherapy, computer-assisted therapy, and educational approaches (e.g., lectures and discussions). Homework assigned to clients can be a key ingredient to successful brief therapy because it makes them take some responsibility for their care. Instead of costly inpatient care, less costly alternatives offering intensive treatment are day treatment, intensive outpatient care, and home care. Community resources such as visiting nurses, self-help groups (e.g., Alcoholics Anonymous, Narcotics Anonymous, Overeaters Anonymous), and vocational and rehabilitation services can also be used. Referral for medication assessment, if appropriate, should occur early in treatment because psychotropic medication may control troublesome symptoms rapidly and thus make the client more accessible to other treatment modalities. Finally, preventive mental health services for groups at risk for developing mental health problems can also be offered to reduce future service use. These might include services for the bereaved, for the newly divorced, for single parents, and for the chronically ill (physical or mental illness), as well as education on predictable life crises (e.g., a child leaving home, retirement, and smoking cessation programs). Because managed-care systems have a vested interest in keeping their members healthy, responding to problems early or preventing them altogether can save considerable time and money.

Attempts to Standardize Treatment

Managed-care systems have reasons to encourage the development and use of clinical decision-making aids (e.g., algorithms and diagnosis-specific treatment protocols). Although these aids are relatively new in mental health care in comparison with physical health care, they are assuming increasing importance. They assist in controlling costs and in promoting quality of care and may be used in utilization review (Grumet, 1988). Algorithms are defined as graphic formats that outline a methodology or prescribed method for diagnosis and treatment. They may assist clinicians in making sound clinical decisions and in providing efficient care (and may thereby protect against claims of negligence), but they may also tend to homogenize care (Grumet, 1988). Research investigating the effects of algorithms on the nature and quality of mental health care apparently does not exist.

Special Concerns

Inpatient Versus Outpatient Care

Although mental health care claims represent an estimated 20–25% of all health care claims, and their number and size are increasing (Developments in the Health Care Marketplace, 1988), in managed-care systems approximately 5% of budgets are typically expended on mental health care, considerably less than expected on the basis of claims experience (Levin, 1988). This may come through controlling inpatient-care costs. Inpatient and residential treatment typically accounts for 75% of all mental health costs (Shulman, 1989). Within inpatient care, substance-abuse and adolescent-psychiatric care account for a large portion of the costs of the typical insurer (Lowman, 1987). As a result, inpatient care, particularly for adolescents and substance abusers, is closely scrutinized by managed-care systems. By avoiding hospitalizations and by decreasing the lengths of psychiatric confinements, costs can also be lowered. Inpatient mental health care can also be controlled in managed systems by precertification of nonemergency admissions, second opinions, and frequent case reviews (Grumet, 1988; Shulman, 1989). Inpatient treatment limitations may also encourage inpatient providers to quickly resort to extreme treatment measures (e.g., electroconvulsive shock therapy) because of the time constraints (Sharfstein, Drunn, & Kent, 1987). Conflicts may arise when inpatient treatment staff do not share the philosophy behind short-term stays and are thus reluctant to alter their treatment strategies. Clients and their families also should be educated about inpatient care so that they have realistic expectations about the probable brief length of stay. Ramsey (1989) suggests that psychiatric emergency room visits be minimized in managed care to avoid client expectations of hospitalization. He also recommends defining hospital-ization as a period of observation so that clients will expect only a brief stay. Because their costs have not been viewed as excessive, outpatient costs have been the source of fewer controls. However, some savings have been realized in outpatient care by matching clients with appropriate therapists and inter-ventions (Berkman et al., 1988).

Care of Chronic Clients

Long-term, chronic mental health care poses special problems for managed health care systems. Many specifically exclude long-term care or care for chronic illness and allow care to be provided to chronically ill clients only when they are undergoing a crisis or experiencing some other type of short-term problem. Yet, this type of client might benefit most from a managed-care approach because psychotherapy alone will seldom adequately address his or her needs. A number of programmatic case-management methods have been devised for such clients (e.g., Community Health Care Plan—Patrick, Coleman, Eagle, & Nelson, 1978; Harvard Health Care—Sabin, 1978). For the care of chronic mental health clients, these methods include frequent (but brief) contact that is pragmatic and problem focused and that includes education as a significant component. Medication management may also be coordinated. In some man-aged-care settings, the benefits of chronically ill clients may be extended to provide them with the services they need, either by increasing the number of prepaid visits, charging copayments only for extra visits, or charging the full fee for additional visits. A survey by Lange et al. (1988) found that all of the HMOs in their study claimed to permit continuation of treatment beyond the maximum number of allowable visits. Alternatively, clients may be transferred to the public sector at the outset of treatment or when benefits have been exhausted if adequate care cannot be provided within the restrictions of the managed-care system (e.g., 20 visits per year). In capitated systems, a financial incentive exists for such transfers.

Resistant or noncompliant clients can cause difficulties for managed-care systems because clients who refuse or do not comply with treatments that are preventive or provide early intervention may develop more severe problems that require more aggressive or more costly treatments. Some HMOs require their clients to sign treatment contracts that state that noncompliance can be grounds for dismissal from the HMO treatment benefit. For example, in the Harvard Community Health Plan, the protocol for noncompliant persons is that noncompliance is first documented in the individual's chart and discussed with the client, then a letter is sent to the client referring to the "termination for cause" section of the member's service contract, and finally, the matter is referred to the medical director, who attempts to meet with the client and family members to discuss the situation and offer possible solutions, with the last resort being termination of the client. Providers in this situation may not be legally at risk because they are following procedure as outlined in the members' service contract, but case law in managed mental health is still emerging (see Newman & Bricklin, chapter 4 in this book).

Organizational Issues

In addition to changing how they practice, clinicians must accept the fact that in managed-care settings their care will be closely monitored not only by business-minded administrators, but by colleagues from their own and other disciplines, quality assurance and utilization review committees, and consumers. Typically, HMOs, PPOs, and other types of managed mental health organizations have utilization review committees and quality-assurance committees, although these are not legal requirements. Less commonly, surveys of client satisfaction may be used as criteria for quality of care. The quality-assurance reviews focus on the appropriateness of care and the degree of client improvement (Bloom, 1987). Utilization review committees pose ethical concerns when their members are drawn exclusively from the managed-care plan's staff, because they may have conflicts of interest if they are also part owners of the organization.

Information management becomes of critical importance in managed systems (Berkman et al., 1988). Typically, the contracting group needs to know at any time its client load, therapist load, and financial health. Data on the client must be tracked from the time of referral until termination. Such tracking relies heavily on clinicians completing intake and progress notes in a timely manner, because they are used to determine the care given and to monitor the case status. Such documentation also facilitates communication among various health care providers involved in the case. Some managed-care systems withhold payment to clinicians until paperwork is turned in, to reinforce the importance of its completion. Data must also be tracked on client copayments if such are collected.

Benefits of Participating in Managed Health Care Systems

Managed health care need not be a negative experience for the practicing clinician. It provides clinicians with opportunities to collaborate with health care professionals from one's own as well as other disciplines, particularly in the staff-model HMO. Because mental health professionals can provide services that reduce the use of physical health care (Mumford, Schlesinger, Glass, Patrick, & Cuerdon, 1984), physicians and other health care providers may welcome their input and involvement. In this manner, psychologists may have the opportunity to become key players on the health care team, rather than isolated practitioners. Such interdisciplinary collaboration may also have drawbacks. In physician-dominated systems, nonphysicians may be expected to collaborate with physicians, yet may be treated as less than equals within the system. Such inequity is not, however, unique to HMOs (e.g., Tulkin & Frank, 1985.)

Clinicians in managed health care settings have already altered some of their working practices. Published reports indicate that a characteristic "HMO therapy" is developing in which the parameters of psychotherapy are being modified to fit the demands and limitations of the setting. Therapists who practice in managed health care settings generally set clearly defined treatment goals rapidly, provide for crisis intervention, schedule sessions flexibly so that their frequency and length are based on client need more than on traditional routine, engage in cooperative interdisciplinary collaboration in treatment planning, work with not only the client, and use a modified version of primary care.

Issues for Clinicians Considering Joining HMOs

Clinicians need to consider carefully the form of managed-care system in which they choose to participate. Evaluation criteria concerning the decision to join or not to join a system include the following:

1. What are the ethical practices of the organization, and is there a demonstrated commitment to provide high-quality services to all clientele?

2. How financially stable is the organization providing the managed care?

3. What has been the staff or contractor turnover rate? (The state insurance board may be able to provide some of this information.)

4. What are the covered mental health benefits, and how are they presented to members?

5. How are chronic illness and specialized needs handled?

6. What roles do quality assurance and utilization review play in the system?

7. Are the quality of the interdisciplinary relationships primarily cooperative or conflictual?

Contractual Arrangements

When clinicians singly or as a group contract to provide mental health services for a managed-care system, other issues should be evaluated before the clinician agrees to participate:

1. Organizationally, does the contracting group have a positive attitude toward providing managed-care services, or is such care viewed as second class? Some settings (and providers) are simply ill suited to managed mental health care because of their philosophy of treatment or personality (see Haas & Cummings, chapter 7 in this book) and probably should not participate.

2. Is there willingness to accept lower fees in return for a potentially larger volume of clients?

3. Clinically and administratively, is the group competent to work with a wide variety of types of people and problems over which clinicians may have little choice or control?

4. Who is responsible for crisis and emergency care and for hospitalization?

General Issues

In establishing an agreement with a specific managed-care organization, it is wise to make provisions in the contract for a variety of issues, many of which are "worst case" scenarios. Explicit elaboration of such issues makes them less likely to occur. Perhaps most important, there must be agreement on what services will be provided, to whom, and under what conditions. Secondly, the agreement should specify how the contractor will be paid. Several common methods of payment are fee for service at the standard, or more typically, discounted rate, holdback, capitation, or payment on a decreasing scale as the number of sessions increases (Berkman et al., 1988).

Generally, contractors are paid by the session (regardless of the amount of time spent) or by the contract. Practitioners should find out whether time paid includes paperwork, telephone calls, and so forth, or face-to-face contact only. (The latter is typical.) Often managed-care systems require their contractors to share financial risk either through capitation or through a holdback system, a notion foreign to many clinicians. Financial survival in a capitated system may depend on the ability to forecast reasonably accurately the amount of mental health care, both inpatient and outpatient, a given population will require. Such forecasting can be done if adequate data exist on the population's characteristics and history of mental health service use and on service-delivery costs. A year or two of experience with the capitated population may be needed before accurate predictions are truly possible. In capitated contexts, the use of inpatient care is of paramount importance because one or two lengthy inpatient stays can easily drain financial resources (see Lowman, chapter 6 in this book). In developing proposals for capitated care, the following risk factors need to be taken into account: number and demographics of covered persons; rate of referral within the covered population; average length of treatment; expected incidence of mental health problems and substance abuse requiring treatment; proportion of referrals requiring specialized services (e.g., crisis intervention, neuropsychological assessment); proportion of referrals requiring inpatient care (psychiatric and substance abuse); average length of inpatient stay; and costs of inpatient providers, outpatient providers, and administrative staff (Cooper, 1989). Copayment collection must also be considered in terms of the amount of money generated and the cost of collecting it. What to do about persons unable to fund the copayment should also be addressed in the contract. Given the current state of HMOs (Shellenbarger, 1990), provisions should also be made concerning what happens if the managed-care system goes bankrupt, including specification of the disposition of clients and whether the contractor is to be paid.

Concerning service-delivery models, the larger practices may wish to create a separate division in the group to perform the contractual work. Such a design allows for specialization with regard to administrative and support staff and makes cost accounting for these services easier. Overhead for managed care may be significantly higher than for a traditional private practice because of information management and more use of administrative and support staff. Multidisciplinary mental health groups may be more attractive to managed-care systems than single-discipline groups because they may offer a broader range of services.

Conclusion

Although there are some constraints when working in managed-care settings, there are also benefits. Psychologists have the opportunity to have an impact on client care by developing new treatment strategies and by testing both old and new interventions. They can work with people throughout the life span and participate in total, rather than traditional piecemeal, health care. Although it appears constraining to the practitioner accustomed to long-term or inpatient treatment, the typical benefit package is in fact adequate for the majority of clients. Of course, there is more to learn, including which persons benefit most from which interventions and under what circumstances, and whether clients who once might have been hospitalized function as well or better without hospitalization. Rather than fighting a probably lost battle by resisting HMOs, clinicians might better learn to work with such systems and contribute to them.

References

Anderson, M. D., & Fox, P. (1987). Lessons learned from Medicaid managed care approaches. *Health Affairs,* spring, 72–86.

Austad, C. S. (1988, October). HMO ideals. *APA Monitor,* p. 2.

Austad, C. S., DeStefano, L., & Kisch, J. (1988). The health maintenance organization: II. Implications for psychotherapy. *Psychotherapy: Theory, Research, and Practice, 25,* 449–454.

Berkman, A. S., Bassos, C. A., & Post, L. (1988). Managed mental health care and independent practice: A challenge to psychology. *Psychotherapy: Theory, Research, and Practice, 25,* 434–440.

Blackwell, B., Gutmann, M., & Gutmann, L. (1988). Case review and quantity of outpatient care. *American Journal of Psychiatry, 145,* 1003–1006.

Bloom, A. (1987). Liability concern of utilization review and quality-assurance programs. *HMO, 1,* 128–133.

Budman, S. (1989, August). *Training experienced clinicians to do brief treatment—Silk purses into sow's ears.* Paper presented at the 97th Annual Convention of the American Psychological Association, New Orleans, LA.

Carr-Kaffashan, L. (1989, August). *Psychologists: Many roles within managed care systems.* Paper presented at the 97th Annual Convention of the American Psychological Association, New Orleans, LA.

Cooper, C. L. (1989, August). Financial management. In L. Richardson (Chair), *Coping with managed mental health care: Transitions in private practice.* Symposium conducted at the 97th Annual Convention of the American Psychological Association, New Orleans, LA.

Cummings, N. (1986). The dismantling of the American health system. *American Psychologist, 41,* 426–431.

Cummings, N. (1988). Emergence of the mental health complex: Adaptive and maladaptive responses. *Professional Psychology, 19,* 308–315.

Cummings, N. A., & Duhl, L. J. (1987). The new delivery system. In L. J. Duhl & N. A. Cummings (Eds.), *The future of mental health services: Coping with crisis* (pp. 87–98). New York: Springer.

Davanloo, H. (1979). Techniques of short-term psychotherapy. *Psychiatric Clinics of North America, 2,* 11–22.

DeLissovoy, G., Rice, T., Gabel, J., & Gelzer, H. J. (1987). Preferred provider organizations one year later. *Inquiry, 24,* 127–135.

Developments in the health care marketplace: A potpourri. (1988, June). *Register Report,* pp. 1, 4, 9–12.

Feldman, S. (1986). Mental health in health maintenance organizations: A report. *Administration in mental health, 13,* 165–179.

Flinn, D. E., McMahon, T. C., & Collins, M. F. (1987). Health maintenance organizations and their implications for psychiatry. *Hospital and Community Psychiatry, 38,* 255–263.

General Accounting Office. (1988). *Medicare physician incentive payments by prepaid health plans could lower quality of care* (GAO/HRD-89-29). Washington, DC: U.S. Government Printing Office.

Goodstein, L. (1986, December 12). Letter to the editor. *The Wall Street Journal,* p. 35.

Grumet, B. R. (1988). The standard of care: Legal considerations in protocols and standing orders. *HMO, 2,* 20–23.

Gurevitz, H. (1984). Psychiatry and preferred provider organizations. *Psychiatric Annals, 14,* 342–349.

Hsia, D. C., Krushat, W., Fagan, A. B., Tebutt, J. A., & Kusserow, R. P. (1988). Accuracy of diagnostic coding for Medicare payment under the prospective payment system. *New England Journal of Medicine, 318,* 352–355.

Hoyt, M. (1985). Therapists' resistance to short-term dynamic psychotherapy. *Journal of the Academy of Psychoanalysis, 13,* 93–112.

Lange, M. A., Chandler-Guy, C., Forti, R., Foster-Moore, P., & Rohman, M. (1988). Providers' views of HMO mental health services. *Psychotherapy: Theory, Research and Practice, 25,* 455–462.

Levin, B. L. (1988). Continued changing patterns in coverage and utilization of mental health, alcohol, and substance abuse within HMOs. *Group Health of America Journal, 8,* 16–28.

Levin, B. L., Glasser, J. H., & Jaffee, C. L. (1988). National trends in coverage and utilization of mental health, alcohol, and substance abuse services within managed health care systems. *American Journal of Public Health, 78,* 1222–1223.

Lowman, R. L. (1987, August). *Economic incentives in the delivery of alternative mental health services.* Paper presented at the 95th Annual Convention of the American Psychological Association, New York, NY.

Mumford, E., Schlesinger, H. J., Glass, G. V., Patrick, C., & Cuerdon, T. (1984). A new look at evidence about reduced cost of medical utilization following mental health treatment. *American Journal of Psychiatry, 141,* 1145–1158.

Pallak, M. (1987, August). *Psychotherapy and public policy (or Daniel enters the lion's den).* Invited address presented at the 95th Annual Convention of the American Psychological Association, New York, NY.

Patrick, D. L., Coleman, J., Eagle, J., & Nelson, E. (1978). Chronic emotional problem patients and their families in an HMO. *Inquiry, 15,* 100.

Phillips, E. L. (1985). *A guide for therapists and patients to short-term psychotherapy.* Springfield, IL: Charles C Thomas.

Phillips, E. L. (1988). Length of psychotherapy and outcome: Observations stimulated by Howard, Kopta, Krause, and Orlinsky. *American Psychologist, 43,* 669–670.

Ramsey, G. (1989, August). *How to manage "managed care"—Meat and potatoes.* Paper presented at the 97th Annual Convention of the American Psychological Association, New Orleans, LA.

Sabin, J. E. (1978). Research findings on chronic mental illness: A model for continuing care in the HMO. *Comprehensive Psychiatry, 19,* 88–95.

Sharfstein, S. S., Drunn, L., & Kent, J. J., Jr. (1987). The clinical consequences of payment limitations: The experience of a private psychiatric hospital. *The Psychiatric Hospital, 19,* 63–66.

Shellenbarger, S. (1990, February 27). As HMO premiums soar, employers sour on the plans and check out alternatives. *The Wall Street Journal,* p. B1.

Shulman, J. (1989, August). *Managed mental health care: Positioning yourself for the future.* Paper presented at the 97th Annual Convention of the American Psychological Association, New Orleans, LA.

Talbott, J. A. (1981). Commentary: The emerging crisis in chronic care. *Hospital and Community Psychiatry, 32,* 447–454.

Tulkin, S. R., & Frank, G. W. (1985). The changing role of psychologists in health maintenance organizations. *American Psychologist, 40,* 1125–1131.

Walworth, J., O'Donnell, P. S., Pearson, J. P., & Solem, E. (1987). *Quality assurance I—What are employers demanding?* Paper presented at the meeting of the Group Health Association of America, Washington, DC.

Zimet, C. N. (1989). The mental health care revolution: Will psychology survive? *American Psychologist, 44,* 703–708.

9

Managed Mental Health Care: Critical Issues and Next Directions

Rodney L. Lowman

For clinicians and researchers alike, managed mental health care presents special challenges. Wise clinicians and observant researchers see opportunities, although others curse unsolicited change. Mental health professionals can be effective players in the current managed mental health care environment, but only if they are informed participants in the managed-care debate. This book is intended to help professionals move from being not very well-informed complainers about the changes they have experienced as the result of the managed-care system to becoming more proactive players in the current managed-care debate. To this end, the contributors to this book have described the present and historical contexts of managed mental health care, have reviewed the current knowledge base, and have suggested ways in which psychologists can better understand managed care and improve its effectiveness. In this concluding chapter, I target the issues that mental health professionals should currently be most proactive in addressing.

Addressing Economic Factors That Affect the Provision of Mental Health Care

As DeLeon, VandenBos, and Bulatao (chapter 2; see also VandenBos, 1993) have shown, the original goal of managed mental health care was to provide affordable, quality care to previously uninsured populations. Although this goal is being met on many levels, some providers, particularly mental health care providers, are finding that cost factors are too often adversely affecting quality of care and that the cost-containment strategies are not founded on empirically derived data.

One especially problematic issue is that of the costs and benefits of inpatient versus outpatient treatment. Although inpatient care accounts for the bulk of mental health care expenditures, there exists no convincing evidence that inpatient care provides a superior result to outpatient care alternatives. I and many others (e.g., Kiesler, 1982a, 1982b; Kiesler & Sibulkin, 1987; Lowman, 1987; chapter 6 in this book) have criticized inpatient mental health

I thank Shirley Ann Higuchi and Gary R. VandenBos for their helpful comments.

care as being largely a scientifically unproved intervention whose efficacy, especially when compared with outpatient alternatives, is far from reliably established. I hope that psychologists will be at the forefront of redefining this all-too-moribund area of practice and research, an area too often influenced more by financial incentives than by scientific research findings (see Lowman, 1987).

Specifically, mental health professionals should consider directing at least as much effort to evaluating the efficacy of inpatient care (versus outpatient alternatives) as they have to the issue of inpatient admission privileges. A better product, at lesser cost, is almost always a more marketable product in a policy arena than is the correction of a perceived injustice. Psychologists and other nonmedically trained professionals may be in a unique position to address this issue because their training and their disciplines have not emerged from medically intensive, hospital-based models.

Another way to approach the cost-versus-quality problem is to recognize that only a small number of a mental health system's users are likely to substantially increase the cost burdens on the system. Managed mental health systems, if they are to prove their overall effectiveness, must be equipped to treat the seriously disturbed as well as those with problems of lesser severity. Such patients are likely to raise cost and care concerns over time, regardless of the nature of the mental health care delivery system. People who are more medically ill naturally consume greater health care resources than those who are less sick, and there is no reason to think that the case is any different with mental health. Presumably no one would argue that patients who are more ill medically should receive identical or less intense interventions than are those less ill. Yet, by analogy, exactly that situation has been applied to mental health care by many managed-care plans.

By excluding those suffering more severe psychological disturbances from any mental health benefit (as is typical in many HMO plans), provider organizations may save immediate costs by shifting these patients outside the managed mental health system, but they are not necessarily meeting the treatment needs of covered patients. In effect, managed-care patients who are denied mental health benefits and who have extensive mental health needs but no money are forced to pay for private care or to seek help in the public sector. It would appear that a criterion for the evaluation of the effectiveness of any managed-care system should be the extent to which the plan effectively addresses the mental health needs of all of its covered lives, including those whose treatment is inevitably more intensive and more expensive than others.

Another problematic economic factor is that the current cost concerns of insurers and third-party payors are at least partly the iatrogenic consequences of mental health benefit design (see chapter 6). Confronted with a mental health crisis and having benefits that pay 100% of inpatient care and 50% or less of outpatient alternatives, financial incentives prevail, at considerable cost to the third-party payors. From a cost-savings perspective, much could be done immediately to lower mental health costs by redesigning mental health benefits to remove the strong incentive toward using costly inpatient care and create incentives for using less expensive outpatient alternatives. The irony is that outpatient psychotherapy, which has abundantly proved its efficacy with rigorous research, is typically given less extensive insurance coverage, whereas inpatient care is often generously funded.

Conducting Research on Cost Versus Outcome

If mental health costs are out of control, it is understandable that cost-containment efforts should be implemented. Although the economic ramifications of untreated mental health problems and the costs associated with different treatment modalities are now well documented, we know considerably less about the interrelationship of managed mental health care costs, utilization of services, and clinical outcomes (Lowman, 1992). A complete evaluation of the effectiveness of managed mental health care cannot be made until substantive, accurate, and long-term outcome data are obtained. The literature is currently deficient in this area. On the whole, managed mental health care should be considered experimental, and, until its effectiveness is established by research, it should be used conservatively and without the assumption of effectiveness. Consider this analogy: It is highly unlikely that any psychopharmaceutical drug would ever have been approved for general consumption with outcome data as scant as the data that exist for managed mental health care outcomes.

Although there are many complex issues that researchers need to explore, answers to the following two questions may yield basic criteria for exploring the cost–outcome relationship of managed mental health care: (a) Overall, do mental health services under managed-care programs cost less than those under traditional models? and (b) Are the immediate and long-term clinical outcomes more or less effective under managed mental health delivery systems? So, for example, given the existing cost patterns, the degree to which managed mental health plans cut inpatient costs without curtailing the benefits of outpatient care may serve as one criterion of a managed-care plan's effectiveness.

Another criterion that may be successfully employed to evaluate effectiveness is the manner in which costs are distributed. Managed mental health care systems often simply change who receives money without changing net costs. Often costs are shifted in order to pay for the administration of health care. Shifting costs to pay high administrative costs can have potentially negative effects on quality of care and clinical outcome. Himmelstein and Woolhandler (1986; Himmelstein, Woolhandler, & the Writing Committee of the Working Group on Program Design, 1989) reported very disturbing statistics about the American form of health care. Woolhandler and Himmelstein (1991) found that administrative expenditures in the United States are 60% higher than in the Canadian health care system and 97% higher than in the British system.

In undertaking research into managed mental health care, it must be recognized that, like mental health hospitalization, managed care is a variably defined intervention that has different meanings depending on what services are managed, who oversees the process, and what outcome evaluation methodology is used. Thus another goal of outcome evaluation research should be to examine the effects of different types of managed care interventions (e.g., alternative benefit plan designs, use of screeners and utilization reviewers, and outpatient treatment incentives) on costs and outcomes. Although there are enthusiastic advocates of managed mental health care models (e.g., Cummings, 1986), some of whom have asserted that most patients can be treated successfully with managed-care methods, more data are needed to identify specifically who is likely to benefit from a particular type of managed mental health care and who may suffer harm. Moreover, this kind of outcome evaluation research can be problematic when, as is common, treatment or reimbursement is subject to several variables at the same time. For example, an entity may decide to redesign benefits, use preadmission screening programs, and limit access to or shorten treatment. Although concerned employers or benefits managers are certainly within their rights to execute changes, when so many variables exist, outcome attributions and generalizations are difficult to make. Under such circumstances, even if cost savings are demonstrated by competently done evaluation research, it may be difficult to determine the source of the apparent savings.

It would be useful, therefore, to review the approach and language of the Health Maintenance Organization Act of 1973, which, although mandating generous (by today's standards) mental health outpatient benefits to enrollees, excluded from mandatory coverage conditions not amenable to short-term care. A comparable medical situation would be to provide generous coverage for acute myocardial infarction but to provide no coverage at all for chronic cardiac conditions. Brief psychotherapy models (the treatment of choice of most managed-care plans) may simply not work for people with certain types of mental health difficulties. To design benefit systems around the one-size-fits-all approach is simplistic, care depriving, and antithetical to the HMO concept of covering all of an individual's health care needs.

Perhaps the greatest potential consequences of managed mental health care have yet to be examined. If uncontrolled access to traditional inpatient mental health care is largely an endangered species, managed health and mental health care are not. The competitive proliferation of managed-care and managed mental health care organizations appears already to have resulted in the existence of fewer, larger organizations that control more and more mental health care (see Cummings, 1988). Larger players have greater control over who provides services and over the types of reimbursible services provided, potentially resulting in larger cost savings, but also in more consolidated power over mental health providers. One consequence may be to decrease costs of mental health care by paying less and less to increasingly controlled providers. Thus, as powerful market or government forces consolidate the number of payors, there may be an incentive to hire fewer and less expensive providers, presumably those with less extensive training. The ultimate result may well be a decline in the quality of mental health services rendered and a significant, unintended impact on who finds the field attractive to enter. As in medicine, where progressively fewer of the most scientifically talented are currently entering the profession, so in the mental health professions the consequences of decreased professional autonomy are likely to be an ultimate decline in the number of aspirants to that profession and in the quality of those who do become mental health practitioners. These potentially serious consequences should not remain unstudied.

Revising Cost-Containment Strategies

Although most readers might agree that certain costly and high-need mental health cases will benefit from some sort of oversight, it is not clear that routine outpatient care requires or benefits from the same intensive scrutiny. If recurring users of inpatient mental health services offer the greatest opportunity for cost containment, it makes little sense to have an elaborate and expensive mental health management scheme controlling psychotherapy sessions in tiny parcels of one to four sessions. The costs of administering such micromanaged plans, although not yet empirically documented, presumably outweigh whatever cost benefit might ensue. For example, greater scrutiny is warranted for a case in which a patient has already been hospitalized twice for substance abuse, has shown no signs of improvement, and is now proposed for a third hospitalization than for a depressed patient who is receiving the allowable 20 sessions of outpatient psychotherapy. Similarly, long-term (defined by some clear and defensible set of criteria) outpatient cases might be a more appropriate focus of careful management and scrutiny than are short-term outpatient cases (see Phillips, 1985, 1988).

Thus, in this alternative mental health benefits model, relatively generous outpatient benefits might be provided to the first-time or periodic user of mental health services, although more closely scrutinized care might occur whenever inpatient services are allegedly needed, or when outpatient care passes some (hopefully empirically defined) threshold point. Such a threshold is no doubt higher than many current managed mental health programs allow. What typically occurs in managed mental health care systems is that referrals of complicated mental health cases are allotted four to six initial outpatient sessions, after which the therapist has to apply, if not to beg, for additional sessions (see also chapter 8 in this book). This practice constitutes neither good psychotherapy nor good case management, so why does it prevail?

First, as I have stated, there is not yet a definitive literature that empirically establishes lengths of treatment versus outcomes for various mental health conditions, leaving a wide-open opportunity for cost management efforts to focus on costs alone. Second, too often a financial incentive exists for mental health systems to use as little mental health care as possible. Such systems attempt to demonstrate their effectiveness by exhibiting lowered costs over some base period. A third reason is that systems offering managed mental health services on a capitated basis may have to underbid in order to get a contract, placing sizable cost conservation pressures on the system. The latter cost pressures are at odds with the spirit and intent of the federal HMO Act, which mandated as a minimal mental health benefit requirement 20 outpatient sessions per client per year.

The curtailment of mental health benefits in managed-care contexts needs further attention in the public policy arena. If, for example, managed-care groups were required to present their annual statistics on mental health utilization, including the average number of sessions used per diagnostic category, potential customers of the managed health system could evaluate with more clarity whether they wished to enroll. Moreover, publishing in a format available to and understandable by the general public the number of case appeals and the direction of the decisions would also help put pressure on the managed-care group not to make arbitrary or overly cost-controlling decisions. Utilization statistics can be powerful in instigating change.

Another partial solution would be to mandate an initial minimal allotment (e.g., 20 sessions) for any patient desiring mental health services, regardless of the mental health condition, which it would then be the referring psychotherapist's responsibility to allocate. Further sessions beyond the initial allotment would then have to be justified and reviewed by a managed-care group. (Inpatient care in such a model could still be very closely scrutinized and rationed.) Alternatively, initial allotments could be authorized by diagnosis, or on some empirical basis, with more serious conditions meriting a larger initial allotment of care. Other benefit designs are also possible, including an increasing copayment as services continue (see chapter 6).

Attending to Legal and Ethical Issues

Inevitably, new forms of practice affect how psychological services are delivered. Newman and Bricklin (chapter 4) and Higuchi (chapter 5) summarized legal, ethical, and professional practice issues attendant to managed mental health care. Haas and Cummings (chapter 7) showed that much work remains to be done to help psychologists behave ethically and responsibly in such settings, particularly when they are not in agreement with externally established treatment parameters. Which type of patient benefits from which type of managed mental health care (if any) is a research and policy question with important ethical implications. Complex forensic and professional practice dilemmas must be considered when clinicians interact with managed-care systems. The thorough review by Higuchi (chapter 5) illustrates that the forensic issues are changing rapidly as case law on managed health care emerges.

The complexity of the medical environment in which managed-care issues are perhaps too often embedded, as several chapters in this book have suggested, necessitates a thorough grounding in legislative realities at the federal and state level if practitioners are to understand how to practice in today's managed-care environment and how to influence that environment. Increasingly complex legal and regulatory environments (Appelbaum, 1993; chapter 5 in this book) define the form that health and mental health benefits will take. Legislation seemingly far removed from the practice of psychology, and often designed to address health policy that is at variance with mental health needs or concerns, too often now dictates mental health practice policy, for better or for worse. Psychological policymakers and practitioners alike need to understand this arena, law by law and case by case. Today, no mental health practitioner can afford to be uninformed on the forensic aspects of mental health care.

As Haas and Cummings (chapter 7) also noted, the practicing clinician must proceed carefully in determining whether he or she has the expertise, if not the temperament, to work within the typical parameters of managed-care systems. Indeed, it may be inappropriate to undertake treatment with a client when the managed-care system's restrictions clearly suggest little chance of a positive outcome or when the required treatment is one that the practitioner does not endorse. At the least, the client must be informed of the parameters of care and, if appropriate, of the clinician's recommendations on what constitutes appropriate care.

Although clinicians may rightfully be concerned about the limited number of therapy sessions being offered to particular clients, the alternative possibility of having no care provided through the insurance plan may be even worse for the well-being of the client. Clinicians may therefore be obliged to appeal decisions made by managed-care groups (Appelbaum, 1993; chapter 5 in this book). Being put in this position poses both an ethical and a legal dilemma for clinicians: Whereas appeals can help protect psychologists from liability, they also may have long-term consequences (e.g., fewer referrals may be made to providers seen as troublemakers, or providers may be dropped without cause from the provider panel).

The practicing clinician wanting to work effectively within managed health contexts, or accurately perceiving that there is no alternative if financial survival is a goal, is left with difficult choices. As Richardson and Austad (chapter 8) noted, managed mental health care from the perspective of today's practicing clinician may be a convoluted, irrational process in which people with limited, if any, mental health training are making clinical decisions about how much and what type of treatment is required. Too often, however, the therapist is left accountable for clinical decisions made by the managed-care system. Clinicians must therefore attend to complex, difficult-to-resolve issues in their interactions with clients whose care is directed by third parties.

One way in which the psychology profession can be proactive in resolving all of the major issues discussed here (i.e., research, cost-containment, legal, and ethical issues) is to ensure that future practitioners are adequately educated. Psychologists and other nonmedical providers have historically had no natural antipathy to cost-efficient mental health treatment, especially that which has demonstrated efficacy. With the noteworthy exception of certain long-term care models of psychotherapy, psychologists have been exemplars of providers of comparatively inexpensive mental health care. Psychologists, as a professional group, cannot be held responsible for excessive mental health costs (although certainly there are some who have abused the systems, particularly in the area of inpatient care).

However, as Broskowski (chapter 1) appropriately noted, clinical and counseling psychologists are not usually trained to function in the modern managed mental health care environment. To train graduate students only in the fineries of conducting long-term, psychodynamically oriented psychotherapy would appear to ill-prepare them for the professional practice they are likely to perform today. It is axiomatic that one cannot teach or practice that which one does not know, and it must be presumed that many faculty are themselves ill prepared to conduct such instruction or, worse, are actively resistant to it.

There are a variety of models of brief therapy and a variety of types of intervention models that fit well within managed mental health settings. Students in the mental health professions need to be exposed both to alternative models of managed health care and to the nature of the practice settings in which they will be likely to spend their careers. The clinical training programs of the future may therefore be advised to train psychologists in brief therapy models, in interacting effectively with managed-care entities, and in legal and professional practice issues associated with utilization review.

Next Directions and Recommendations

A common theme of all of the chapters in this book is that, like it or not, managed mental health care is here to stay. Not all psychologists welcome it, but, as Broskowski (chapter 1) demonstrated, the environmental context in which managed health care has been incubated has raised cost consciousness (see also Davis, Anderson, Rowland, & Steinberg, 1990; Frank, 1993; VandenBos, 1993). Third-party payors and employers are simply no longer willing simply to pass along mental health benefits costs without scrutinizing how their insured's money is being spent and how to manage mental health expenditures more carefully.

There seems to be little doubt that the managed aspects of mental health have to date largely been cost driven, and managers have approached cost containment as yet another income-generating activity rather than as a means of balancing the needs of the multiple shareholders of the system (consumers, payors, government, etc.). At least as important as cost is the issue of quality of outcome. (Some, presumably those not paying the bills, would argue that quality concerns surpass cost factors.) Although quality issues have yet to be adequately addressed in the literature, cost savings obtained at the expense of quality impose obvious limitations on the provision of mental health care services. However, the same issues of quality of outcome apply to traditional forms of care, which, especially in the case of inpatient care, have been examined in less detail than might be assumed, and seldom with positive conclusions about the effectiveness of the intervention (see Kiesler & Sibulkin, 1987; chapter 6 in this book). The costs of losing effective providers to other disciplines should also be considered.

Most welcome to the future debates about managed care will be those with clear, convincing, replicable data on the effects, intended and unintended, of managed mental health care on both costs and quality of care. Until well-designed studies are completed, however, policy decisions can and will be made on the basis of current knowledge and assumption. Based on what is currently known, I offer the following recommendations.

1. *The nature and relative efficacy of alternative approaches to the management of mental health costs need to be identified.* Although managed health care firms, which have an obvious economic vested interest in outcomes, publish cost–outcome data in their marketing literature, these data are not supported by literature that would meet even minimally acceptable scientific standards, nor have studies generally been conducted by professionals from outside the system. Moreover, the typical intervention is multifaceted, so that it is difficult to determine whether any alleged cost savings are attributable to benefit redesign, preadmission screening, second-opinion programs, or some combination thereof. Employers and third-party payors should insist on (and pay for) competent external evaluation of managed mental health care intervention efforts so that they will know, as they now cannot, whether such interventions are effective. At the least, before-and-after studies should be conducted.

Descriptions and evaluations of the various types of managed health care models need to be much more detailed. Cost-containment programs often make a number of changes simultaneously. If such systems are effective in reducing costs, it is subsequently difficult to determine the source of the positive outcomes and to replicate the findings in other settings. "Managed mental health care" is not a defined variable or intervention. Presumably, different interventions (e.g., benefit redesign, preadmission screening, and concurrent case management) will be called for in different types of settings (e.g., inpatient versus outpatient) and for different types of populations (e.g., child or adult or chronic versus situationally disturbed). The model I describe (see chapter 6) for analyzing mental health claims may be useful for determining which types of issues need special attention and planning in a given insured population. The model also has relevance for evaluating the effectiveness of intervention programs on targeted problem areas.

Until managed care itself is properly defined and evaluated, it should be considered an experimental method whose costs and consequences (intended and unintended) are unknown. At least as much research attention should be directed to the economic and clinical effectiveness of managed mental health care systems as to mental health care services themselves.

2. *Mental health benefit design should be carefully studied and evaluated.* Excessive mental health benefits costs may largely be a function of inappropriate benefit design. Although research on utilization rates under different benefit plans has been conducted (e.g., McCall & Rice, 1983; Schlesinger, Mumford, Glass, Patrick, & Sharfstein, 1983), generally suggesting that mental health utilization is relatively constant regardless of the benefit design, such studies need to be replicated in light of new benefit packages such as those discussed in chapter 6. When implemented in practice, these plans need to be evaluated to determine both cost and quality outcomes. Having a baseline and continual access to mental health claims experience data greatly facilitates this process.

Whatever the benefit design, the major costs of mental health care in this country continue to be expended on inpatient care, typically estimated to account for 75% or more of the overall mental health costs (Mosher, 1983). In the private sector, advertising and marketing costs heavily influence the costs of inpatient treatment, along with all of the per diem and professional service charges that are associated with hospital stays. Although unstudied in the professional literature, one would reasonably expect that heavy advertising and marketing costs contribute to high costs of inpatient care in the private sector. Because consumers and third-party payors ultimately pay for such marketing efforts, at the least mental health facilities might, as part of their licensing requirements, be mandated to disclose the amount that they expend on such services each year. For faster control of this phenomenon, the hospital accrediting associations might also address these issues.

Pending research findings that warrant otherwise, mental health benefits should be redefined to reflect what is known about the efficacy of various treatment interventions. Outpatient mental health treatment has been the subject of literally thousands of studies demonstrating its generic effectiveness (e.g., Cummings & Failed, 1976; DeLeon, VandenBos, & Cummings, 1983; Parloff, 1982; Smith, Glass, & Miller, 1980). This research suggests that outpatient benefits can and should be liberalized, just as inpatient care benefits can significantly be reduced. The track record of research-verified efficacy of outpatient psychotherapy is well established indeed, and while there can be no presumption that more care is better care (see chapter 6), clearly the greatest potential for cost containment lies with inpatient, not outpatient, mental health care. That is not to say that there should be no containment of outpatient costs, but rather that there is far more need to curtail inpatient than outpatient expenditures.

3. *The consequences of employing large pools of providers need to be evaluated carefully.* Currently, there is a strong movement afoot to combine providers into megapools, which then presumably can better be controlled from a cost-of-care standpoint (see Daschle, Cohen, & Rice, 1993). There is at least one potential consequence other than cost savings that warrants close scrutiny. If a small number of firms control access to patients, particularly if the pools are created in the private sector (Bingaman, Frank, & Billy, 1993), consolidation of power may ultimately serve to lessen, not increase, competition. Provider-pool consolidation appears already to be happening in the mergers of managed-care entities into fewer but larger groups that control more of the mental health market. Such groups currently can exclude highly qualified providers simply because their pools are reported by them to be full. The net effect of such arrangements is, potentially, to allow the consolidation of power in the allocation of mental health resources and increasingly to dictate how mental health care will be delivered and by whom. Those few mental health providers who are credentialed early on in the process, or those who, although having lesser qualifications, are willing to perform the services more cheaply, may be given the majority of the patients. Providers included in panels may be reluctant to confront the system or challenge current practices for fear of losing their favored status.

Conclusion

Overall, managed mental health care has, as of this writing, not yet proved its effectiveness. Mental health professionals must for now work within these systems, which with little effort could be made more effective. The burden of proving the long-term effectiveness of managed mental health care rests with its advocates and promoters.

References

Appelbaum, P. S. (1993). Legal liability and managed care. *American Psychologist, 48,* 251–257.

Bingaman, J., Frank, R. G., & Billy, C. L. (1993). Combining a global health budget with a market-driven delivery system: Can it be done? *American Psychologist, 48,* 270–276.

Cummings, N. A. (1986). The dismantling of our health system: Strategies for the survival of psychological practice. *American Psychologist, 41,* 426–431.

Cummings, N. A. (1988). Emergence of the mental health complex: Adaptive and maladaptive responses. *Professional Psychology: Research and Practice, 19,* 308–315.

Cummings, N. A., & Failed, W. T. (1976). Brief psychotherapy and medical utilization: An eight year follow-up. In H. Dorken & Associates (Eds.), *The professional psychologist today: New developments in law, health insurance, and health practice* (pp. 165–174). San Francisco: Jossey-Bass.

Daschle, T. A., Cohen, R. J., & Rice, C. L. (1993). Health-care reform: Single-payer models. *American Psychologist, 48,* 265–269.

Davis, K., Anderson, G. F., Rowland, D., & Steinberg, E. P. (1990). *Health care cost containment.* Baltimore: Johns Hopkins University Press.

DeLeon, P. H., VandenBos, G. R., & Cummings, N. A. (1983). Psychotherapy—Is it safe, effective and appropriate? The beginning of an evolutionary dialogue. *American Psychologist, 38,* 907–911.

Frank, R. G. (1993). Health-care reform: An introduction. *American Psychologist, 48,* 258–260.

Health Maintenance Organization Act of 1973, Sections 280(c), 300(e)(1)(b), 300(e)(1)(c)–(6)(a), 300(e)(1)(d), 42 U.S.C. (1987).

Himmelstein, D. W., & Woolhandler, S. (1986). Cost without benefit: Administrative waste in U.S. health care. *New England Journal of Medicine, 314,* 441–445.

Himmelstein, D. W., Woolhandler, S., & the Writing Committee of the Working Group on Program Design. (1989). A national health program for the United States: A physician's proposal. *New England Journal of Medicine, 320,* 102–108.

Kiesler, C. A. (1982a). Mental hospitals and alternative care: Noninstitutionalization as potential public policy for mental patients. *American Psychologist, 37,* 349–360.

Kiesler, C. A. (1982b). Public and professional myths about mental hospitalization. *American Psychologist, 37,* 1323–1339.

Kiesler, C., & Sibulkin, A. (1987). *Mental hospitalization: Myths and facts about a national crisis.* Newbury Park, CA: Sage.

Lowman, R. L. (1987, August–September). *Economic incentives in the delivery of alternative mental health services.* Paper presented at the annual meeting of the American Psychological Association, New York, NY.

Lowman, R. L. (1992). Managing mental health care wisely: More is not necessarily better. *Professional Psychology, 23,* 164–166.

McCall, N., & Rice, T. (1983). A summary of the Colorado clinical psychology/expanded mental health benefits experiment. *American Psychologist, 38,* 1279–1291.

Mosher, L. R. (1983). Alternatives to psychiatric hospitalization: Why has research failed to be translated into practice? *New England Journal of Medicine, 309,* 1579–1580.

Parloff, M. B. (1982). Psychotherapy research evidence and reimbursement decisions. *American Journal of Psychiatry, 139,* 718–727.

Phillips, E. L. (1985). *A guide for therapists and patients to short-term psychotherapy*. Springfield, IL: Charles C Thomas.

Phillips, E. L. (1988). Length of psychotherapy and outcome: Observations stimulated by Howard, Kopta, Krause, and Orlinsky. *American Psychologist, 43*, 669–670.

Schlesinger, H. J., Mumford, E., Glass, G. V., Patrick, C., & Sharfstein, S. (1983). Mental health treatment and medical care utilization in a fee-for-service system: Outpatient mental health treatment following the onset of a chronic disease. *American Journal of Psychiatry, 141*, 1145–1158.

Smith, M. L., Glass, G. V., & Miller, T. I. (1980). *The benefits of psychotherapy*. Baltimore: Johns Hopkins University Press.

VandenBos, G. R. (1993). U.S. mental health policy: Proactive evolution in the midst of health care reform. *American Psychologist, 48*, 283–290.

Woolhandler, S., & Himmelstein, D. W. (1991). The deteriorating administrative efficiency of the U.S. health care system. *New England Journal of Medicine, 324*, 1253–1258.

Author Index

Page numbers in italics refer to listings in reference sections.

Subject Index

Claims analysis
  in cost-containment strategies, 7
  data needs in mental health care, 129–130
  of employer's expenditures, in case study,
    119–125
  individual utilization patterns, 125–129
  as management tool, 119
Competitive medical plans, 49
Complaint resolution
  in HMOs, 94
  for psychologists in managed care, 111–112
  in utilization review process, 85, 86
Compliance issues, 58
Concurrent review, 11
Confidentiality
  claims investigation and, 115
  in HMOs, 94
  legal liability in, 101–102
  in managed care settings, 57
  in PPO regulation, 90
  in utilization review process, 85, 86
Consumer protection
  in preferred provider arrangements, 87, 89–
    90
  in state regulation of HMOs, 93–94
  in utilization review legislation, 86
Consumer understanding, 34–35, 68
  of benefit design, 113–116, 147
  of financial incentive plans, 72–73, 74–75,
    89, 93–94, 100
  mental health care utilization statistics for,
    174
  of organization as provider of care, 97–98
  psychology profession's role in, 81
Continuity of care, 10
  legal issues in, 101
Contracts
  concerns of psychologists in, 110–111, 112
  evaluation criteria for psychologists, 142–
    143, 163–164
  hold-harmless provisions in, 102–104
  marketing materials as, 98, 105
  monitoring of therapy sessions by managed
    care organization in, 102
  no-cause terminations and, 106, 108–110
  patient noncompliance in, 161
  psychologist as independent provider, 51–
    52
  psychologist compensation in, 164
  psychologists' concerns with, 55, 104–105,
    155
Corcoran v. United Health Care, 95–96
Cost of care
  advertising/marketing component of, 178
  benefit design and, 119, 130–131, 170–171,
    173–174
  cause of increases in, 3–5, 63

  in CHAMPUS, 25
  claims analysis and, 129–130
  containment strategies, 5–7, 41
  effectiveness of managed care systems, 12–
    14, 35–36
  employer expenditures on, case study of,
    119–125
  high-utilization consumers, 5, 125–129, 131
  individual expenditures, 3
  inpatient vs. outpatient services, 131–133,
    134–135, 140, 141–142, 160–161, 169–
    170
  legal liability in containment strategies,
    70–72
  mental health benefits in HMO plans, 31–
    32
  as percentage of gross national product, 2,
    42
  in PPOs, 46–47
  profession of psychology and, 37
  provider compensation and containment of,
    110–111
  quality of care and, 51, 64, 74, 80–81
  research needs, 171–173, 177
  trends in, 1–3, 8–11, 42, 139–140
Credentialing, legal liability in, 73–74, 98
Crisis intervention
  admissions procedures, 56–57
  in employee assistance programs, 47
  in psychologist–HMO contracts, 52
  in staff model HMOs, 56

Darling v. Charleston Community Memorial
  Hospital, 73
Defense, Department of. See CHAMPUS
Depressive disorders
  reimbursement system as factor in assess-
    ment of, 37, 64
  treatment setting as factor in assessment
    of, 36–37
Diagnostic and Statistical Manual of Mental
  Disorders (DSM-III-R), 58
Diagnostic related groupings
  data collection in claims analysis, 130
  introduction of, 3, 5
  mental disorders in, 9

EAPs. See Employee assistance programs
Emergency admissions, 56–57
Employee assistance programs (EAPs)
  characteristics of, 47–49
  marketing activities in, 55–56
  psychologist ownership of, 51
  psychologists in, 52–53, 53–54
  role of, 47, 48
Employee Retirement Income Security Act of
  1974 (ERISA), 8, 66, 96, 100, 107

About the Editors

Rodney L. Lowman is founder and CEO of The Development Laboratories, Houston, Texas, which offers psychological assessment and counseling on career, work, and mental health issues. He is also an adjunct professor of psychology at Rice University and has served on the faculty of Duke University Medical Center's occupational medicine and medical psychology divisions. Dr. Lowman has written widely on mental health in the workplace and on occupational and career issues. He also consults to national media. He has served on the American Psychological Association's (APA) Ethics Committee, as chair of the APA's Board of Professional Affairs, and as president of the Society of Psychologists in Management. Currently, he serves on the APA's Committee on Psychological Tests and Assessments.

Robert J. Resnick, the 1995 APA president, is a professor of psychiatry and pediatrics, as well as chair of the Division of Clinical Psychology at the Health Sciences Center, Medical College of Virginia, Virginia Commonwealth University. He is a diplomate in clinical psychology of the American Board of Professional Psychology, an APA fellow, past chair of the APA Board of Professional Affairs, past chair of the Association for the Advancement of Psychology, a member of the APA Board of Directors, and past president of the APA Division of Independent Practice. Dr. Resnick was a member of one and the chair of three APA task forces on hospital practice, advocacy, credentialing, and alternative health delivery systems. He has published widely in the area of public policy and psychological practice and has testified before Congress on national health proposals.